Brain Imaging in Epilepsy

Published by the Remedica Group

Remedica Publishing, 32–38 Osnaburgh Street, London, NW1 3ND, UK
Remedica Inc, 20 N Wacker Drive, Suite 1642, Chicago, IL 60606, USA

E-mail: books@remedica.com
www.remedica.com

Publisher: Andrew Ward
In-house editor: Roisin O'Brien

ISBN 1 901346 24 2
British Library Cataloguing-in Publication Data
A catalogue record for this book is available from the British Library

Brain Imaging in Epilepsy

David D Maudgil

Department of Radiology
Royal Free Hospital
London
UK

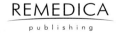

REMEDICA
publishing

LONDON • CHICAGO

For Veenu, Uday and Megha,
with love

Acknowledgements

I would like to thank many people for their help: Professor Simon Shorvon for stimulating my interest in neurology, Professor John Duncan for his comments on the manuscript and writing the foreword, Dr John Buscombe for reviewing the manuscript, Professor Isky Gordon, Drs Alex Hammers, Mark Symms, and Mary McLean at the National Society of Epilepsy, Andrea Kassner at Philips Medical for providing illustrations, Dr Ian Francis for helping me get started, and all the staff at Remedica, especially Roisin O'Brien and Andrew Ward, for their patience and professionalism.

Foreword

Epilepsy is the most common serious neurological disease, with a cumulative lifetime incidence of 1 in 30. Great strides have been made in brain imaging over the last decade and this has improved our understanding of the causes and consequences of the epilepsies, which has aided clinical decision-making. Structural imaging with MRI will commonly reveal the structural basis of partial seizures. Functional imaging, however, can demonstrate the pathophysiological processes that occur in epilepsy. The traditional isotopic methods of PET and SPECT continue to be useful, particularly for ligand studies. It is, however, MRI-based techniques that have developed enormously over recent years, with the advantages of versatility and non-reliance on ionizing radiation. Trained as a Radiologist, but with a background in clinical and research work in epilepsy, and particularly in brain imaging, David Maudgil is in an ideal position to review this fast-moving and fascinating field.

John Duncan MA, DM, FRCP
Medical Director, National Society for Epilepsy
Professor of Neurology, UCL, UK

Contents

CHAPTER 1
Epilepsy

Clinical significance of epilepsy

Epilepsy is the most common serious neurological condition (see **Table 1.1**). Currently, in the developed world, approximately one person in every 50 suffers one or more afebrile seizure during their lifetime, and one person in 200, i.e. 2.3 million people in the US and 350,000 people in the UK, suffers from chronic epilepsy [1–3]. It is estimated that there are 181,000 people in the US diagnosed with new-onset epilepsy every year [3]. People with epilepsy have an increased morbidity rate and they suffer social and psychological handicap [1]; epilepsy makes a 9% contribution to the total socioeconomic burden resulting from neurological and mental disease, and is second only to depression.

Table 1.1. The frequency of neurological disorders. Data from Bradley WG, Daroff RB, Fenichel GM et al., editors. *Neurology in Clinical Practice.* 3rd edition. Boston: Butterworth-Heinemann, 2000.

Neurological disorder	Number of cases per 100,000 people
Epilepsy	650
Acute stroke	600
Dementia	250
Parkinson's disease	200
Multiple sclerosis	60
Motor neuron disease	6
Malignant brain tumor	5

People with epilepsy secondary to another pathology, such as a brain tumor or cerebrovascular disease, have a higher standardized mortality rate (SMR) than would be expected from the underlying pathology alone. Retrospective community studies have indicated an SMR 2- to 3-fold higher than the rate observed in the general population [4], and nearly 4-fold higher in the first 10 years after diagnosis. Clinic-based populations have a higher mortality rate, although this may be because these patients tend to have more complicated conditions and more severe epilepsy. A study of 601 patients attending an epilepsy clinic in 1990 revealed an SMR of 4.5 [5]. Patients with additional neurological problems, such as learning difficulties, have even higher SMRs – as high as 15.9 [6].

Care for people with epilepsy is expensive, since 10% of all epilepsy patients will require institutional care and 60% will require regular medical attention. In the US, these proportions represent 230,000 and 1.4 million people, respectively [7], and it is estimated that the annual cost for prevalent cases is $12.5 billion. The lifetime cost for all people with new-onset epilepsy that are diagnosed within 1 year is $11.1 billion [3].

Table 1.2. Characteristics of patients in the National General Practice Study of Epilepsy (NGPSE) (N=1,195) [13].

Patient characteristics	Number of cases
Excluded	104
Febrile convulsions	220
Nonepileptic	79
Possible epilepsy	228
Definite epilepsy	564
Idiopathic/cryptogenic	346 (61%)
Remote symptomatic	119 (21%)
Acute symptomatic	83 (15%)
Associated with neurological deficit	16 (3%)

The socioeconomic outcome of epilepsy is more difficult to quantify, with previous studies recognizing that up to 75% of patients with epilepsy have problems with employment [8,9]. Studies have also demonstrated that patients with epilepsy, if employed, generally have less skilled jobs, although this may be because they tend to leave school with lower qualifications than average [10]. Approximately half of patients complain of discrimination at work because of their epilepsy [11].

Causes of epilepsy

Knowing the cause of a patient's epilepsy helps in the determination of an optimal therapy. Different epilepsy syndromes (discussed further in Chapter 3) have different treatment strategies, e.g. sodium valproate is thought to be the best treatment for juvenile myoclonic epilepsy, whereas carbamazepine is probably the best treatment for temporal lobe epilepsy. Moreover, knowing the underlying etiology is useful for determining the likely prognosis [12]. In various populations, many studies have attempted to determine the causes of epilepsy. Variation in factors such as the age of the population [13], the geographical location [14], and the availability of high-resolution neuroimaging techniques have suggested a wide range of causes.

Hospital-based series, although plentiful, are considerably hampered by selection bias, since cases that reach hospital neurology clinics are likely to be more severe, chronic, and unrepresentative of the true situation in the general population. The findings of one series, the National General Practice Study of Epilepsy (NGPSE), produced by the National Hospital of Neurology and Neurosurgery in London, are provided in **Table 1.2**. The NGPSE study overcame the limitation of only including clinic-based patients by carrying out a population-based, cohort study of 1,195 patients with newly diagnosed or suspected epileptic seizures [13]. Patients with definite afebrile epileptic seizures were separated into three main groups (see **Table 1.2**):

Table 1.3. The etiology of epilepsy in the National Society of Epilepsy Magnetic Resonance Imaging Study (NSE-MRI). The data are courtesy of Dr A Everitt, National Society of Epilepsy.

Etiology	Newly diagnosed epilepsy	Chronic active epilepsy
Cryptogenic	25%	40%
Cerebrovascular disease	29%	9%
Idiopathic generalized epilepsy	15%	8%
Hippocampal sclerosis	2%	17%
Degenerative disease	10%	2%
Tumors	8%	2%
Head trauma	4%	6%
Birth asphyxia	2%	7%
Malformations of cortical development (recognized on 2-dimensional imaging)	1%	2%

- remote symptomatic – with central nervous system lesions acquired postnatally, which are "remote" in time from the onset of epilepsy
- acute symptomatic – seizures starting within 3 months of an acute insult, such as head trauma or stroke, or associated with a congenital or perinatal neurological abnormality
- cryptogenic – including idiopathic generalized epilepsy (IGE) and those patients with no known predisposing cause

Although comprehensive, the NGPSE study was limited by the absence of magnetic resonance (MR) scanning, which only became widely available in the latter part of the 1990s. The National Society of Epilepsy Magnetic Resonance Imaging (NSE-MRI) study, which was initiated in 1995, was able to take advantage of this diagnostic technique. NSE-MRI was a community-based study including a total population of 200,000 in the South of England in which all patients with epilepsy, or possible epilepsy, were investigated by clinical interview, electroencephalography (EEG), and MR scanning. Preliminary data from the study, indicating the etiology of epilepsy, are provided in **Table 1.3.** It is important to note that, in this study, IGE was classified as a separate condition from cryptogenic epilepsy.

The inclusion of MR imaging as part of the NSE-MRI study meant that more causes for epilepsy could be identified (in particular cerebrovascular disease); therefore, fewer patients than in the NGPSE study were diagnosed as cryptogenic. Nonetheless, a substantial proportion of patients with cryptogenic epilepsy were still identified (up to 40% in the chronic epilepsy group). These individuals constitute a group of patients who are most intractable to treatment, not least because often there is no clear rationale for therapy. Improved diagnosis of the cause of cryptogenic epilepsy will significantly influence the medical management of large numbers of patients.

Chronicity of epilepsy

In the past, patients with epilepsy have been unjustifiably labeled with a pessimistic prognosis. In 1881, Gowers, who has considerably influenced the neurological establishment, stated that: "the spontaneous cessation of the disease (epilepsy) is an event too rare to be reasonably anticipated in any given case" [15]. In 1968, Rodin reinforced this idea by describing epilepsy as a: "chronic condition characterized by a tendency to seizure relapse" [16]. These observations were probably based on studies of hospital patients, who generally have more severe epilepsy and other associated neurological problems.

These ideas were overturned with the advent of population-based studies, such as those performed by the Rochester, Minnesota group, which showed that up to 76% of patients achieved long-term remission [17]. Another community-based study in Tonbridge in the UK also demonstrated that more than two thirds of patients entered remission [18]. Previous epidemiological studies support these findings, indicating that, although 2%–5% of people suffer from epilepsy at some point in their life, at any one time only 0.5% will have epilepsy [4,19,20].

Further studies have confirmed that, in up to 70% of patients, seizures will remit spontaneously or be controlled with medical therapy [12,21]. However, the remaining 30% will continue to have seizures despite all medical treatments, and will eventually be classified as having chronic epilepsy (defined as regular seizures for 5 or more years). Considerable costs are incurred by the patient in terms of increased morbidity and mortality. The social and economic implications to both the patient and the carer are also great. The majority of epilepsy-associated burdens are due to the chronic form of the condition.

The neurophysiological basis of epilepsy

As investigative techniques have become progressively more sophisticated, our understanding of the neurophysiological basis of epilepsy has expanded so that we now have a scientific model for the changes that occur at the cellular level before, during, and after an epileptic seizure.

Functional brain changes before, during, and after the epileptic ictus

These changes will be described to illustrate the theoretical basis for contrast generation in functional images.

Electrical changes

Electrical changes are detected using EEG, which is widely available and is a commonly performed investigation in patients with epilepsy. Although it is an important diagnostic tool, EEG has significant limitations. Since this technique is only a surface recording, there is considerable blurring and attenuation of the brain's electrical activity, and for practical purposes surface electrodes only measure the activity arising from an area of several cm^2 of cerebral cortex underneath them [23].

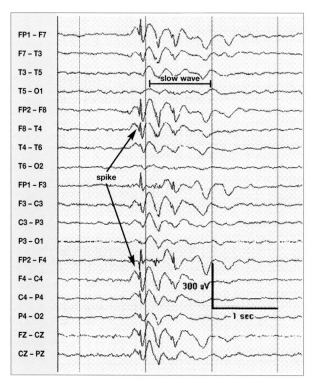

Figure 1.1. Electroencephalogram recording showing a spike and slow wave.

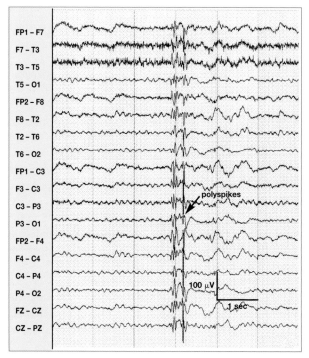

Figure 1.2. Electroencephalogram recording showing generalized polyspikes.

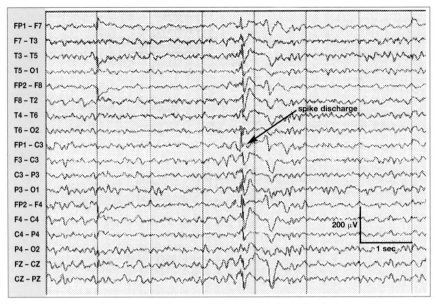

Figure 1.3. Electroencephalogram recording showing a single generalized spike discharge.

Interictal changes

The most common epileptiform abnormalities found in interictal EEG recordings are:

- spikes – an abrupt change in electrical discharge lasting less than 80 ms
- sharp waves – an abrupt change in electrical discharge lasting between 80–120 ms
- spike-wave complex – a spike followed by a slow wave of duration greater than 120 ms

Examples of spikes and slow waves, generalized polyspikes, and a single generalized spike discharge are provided in **Figures 1.1, 1.2,** and **1.3**, respectively.

These abnormalities are "epileptiform", since, although they are commonly observed in patients with epilepsy, they may also be identified in individuals with no history of the disease; hence, they are suggestive – but not diagnostic – of epilepsy.

Spikes and sharp waves both arise from excessive and hypersynchronous excitatory neural activity, which is a direct result of irritation by a lesion. The spike-wave complex is a combination in which the spike comes from excitatory activity in the superficial cortical layer and the slow wave is probably due to inhibitory activity in a deeper layer (because of differing patterns of ionic shift, both signals appear to have the same polarity).

In partial epilepsies, the interictal epileptiform abnormalities appear fairly closely related to the location of the epileptogenic lesion; they appear in the irritative zone. This zone is not observed in generalized epilepsies. As the epileptic ictus is about to begin, spikes and sharp waves build up in amplitude and frequency in a wider area

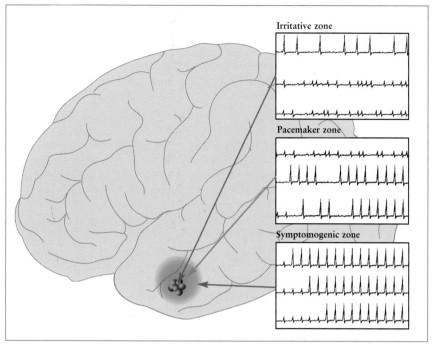

Figure 1.4. A schematic illustration of the spatial and electrographic relationships between the irritative, pacemaker, and symptomogenic zones.

around the irritative zone, known as the pacemaker zone. This zone may not be seen in generalized epilepsies, which tend to start with widespread ictal activity and no obvious localization. The spatial and electrographic relationships between the irritative, pacemaker, and symptomogenic zones are illustrated schematically in **Figure 1.4** and are discussed more fully in the following section.

Ictal changes
Once the ictus has been established, there are widespread synchronized discharges. The locus of electrographic abnormality is the symptomogenic zone. This represents the cortical area affected during the ictus, which will give rise to the clinical symptoms manifested during a seizure.

In generalized epilepsies, the EEG pattern may be:

- a spike and wave (see **Figure 1.5**)
- fast-wave activity
- a diffuse electrodecremental response – a generalized decrease in wave amplitude (see **Figure 1.6**)
- a generalized slow wave, predominantly in the frontal regions

In focal epilepsies, similar patterns may be observed, although the electrical discharge usually does not spread over such a wide area, which accounts for the clinical signs of the seizure that are observed (see Chapter 4).

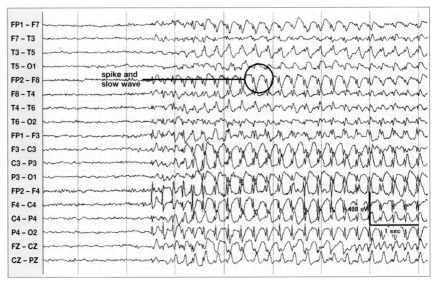

Figure 1.5. Electroencephalogram recording of a spike and wave complex.

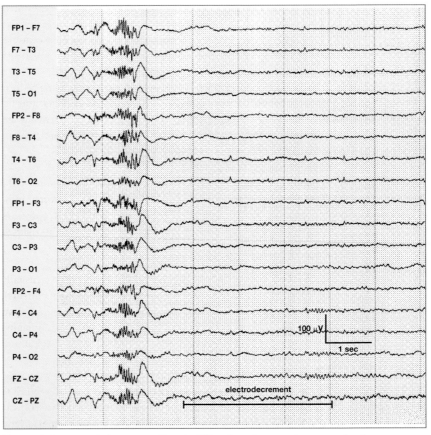

Figure 1.6. Electroencephalogram recording of a diffuse electrodecremental response after sharp waves.

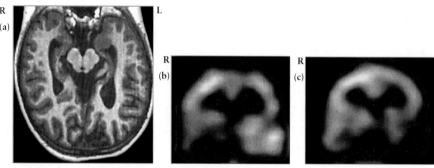

Figure 1.7. Right hippocampal sclerosis: (a) magnetic resonance imaging scan; (b) interictal SPECT showing right temporal hypoperfusion; (c) ictal SPECT showing right temporal hyperfusion. L: left; R: right; SPECT: single photon emission computed tomography. This figure is courtesy of Professor I Gordon.

Blood flow and metabolism

Interictal changes

Typically, structural lesions are surrounded by an area of hypometabolism with decreased blood flow and glucose utilization (see **Figure 1.7**). This is thought to be caused by deafferentation (a decline in neuronal excitement) or active inhibition of the surrounding neural tissue by the lesion. This is supported by the observation that hypometabolism in the remaining temporal lobe cortex gradually normalizes after selective amygdalo-hippocampectomy (surgical removal of the amygdalo-hippocampal complex in the mesial temporal lobe) for the treatment of hippocampal sclerosis causing temporal lobe epilepsy [24]. The study of cavernomas (cavernous hemangiomas) provides additional supporting data. Cavernomas have a surrounding hypometabolic area; the size of this area is unrelated to the size of the underlying lesion. This implies that the hypometabolism is a consequence of alterations of metabolism in the locus surrounding the lesion, rather than the physical effect (such as pressure) exerted by it. Also, the degree of hypometabolism induced by the lesion correlates well with the relief obtained after surgery.

The area of hypometabolism is usually extensive when compared to the size of the lesion, presumably because a functional pathway in close proximity is affected in its entirety. Occasionally, the structural lesion may be much larger than the area of hypometabolism, although in these cases the epileptic focus is always found within the hypometabolic area [25].

In patients with frontal lobe epilepsy, blood flow changes, if they occur, are usually a result of hypometabolism (these changes occur in approximately 60% of patients). A lesion is demonstrated in about 90% of cases. With this form of epilepsy, metabolic changes are more subtle than changes observed by structural imaging techniques [25,26].

Some children with partial seizures show areas of increased metabolism associated with regions of spike-wave abnormality on EEG. The increased metabolism and EEG activity are thought to arise in areas of focal thickening in the cortex, which is probably due to local areas of developmental malformation. In generalized epilepsy, studies have not as yet shown consistent changes in interictal blood flow and metabolism.

Ictal changes

Changes in blood flow occur more slowly than changes in electrical activity (over a few seconds, rather than tenths of seconds). Partial seizures are associated with increased glucose utilization and local blood flow in the affected area with decreases elsewhere [27,28]. Absence epilepsy is associated with a 15% increase in cerebral blood flow and a more modest increase in thalamic blood flow. This correlates with the current view that spike-wave activity in absence attacks is due to oscillating electrical activation in thalamocortical circuits [29].

Neurotransmitter function

The timescale of changes in neurotransmitter expression and binding is many orders of magnitude greater than the timescale of changes previously described. Therefore, the study of these neurotransmitter changes is particularly useful for comparing steady-state differences between patients with epilepsy and controls.

Increased binding to central benzodiazepine receptors (cBZRs) has been reported in patients with IGE [30]. In contrast, in other studies, no increased binding in the cerebral cortex or thalamus was found in patients with absence epilepsy (not being treated with sodium valproate) compared with controls. However, in these patients, a smaller volume of distribution was observed, implying a reduced concentration of cBZRs [31]. Abnormal binding patterns have also been demonstrated in patients with cortical development malformations, which reflect an underlying abnormal distribution of gray matter in the cortex [32].

Conclusion

Epilepsy is an important and common condition that affects millions of people worldwide. By improving our understanding of the causes of epilepsy, we can increasingly offer improved therapies, which will enable patients to enjoy a significantly higher standard of health. Recent advances in our knowledge of the neurophysiological and neurochemical basis of epilepsy are particularly encouraging. In Chapter 2, the latest structural and functional imaging techniques are described. Identifying areas of altered neurophysiology and neurochemistry will allow us to diagnose and locate abnormalities and, therefore, plan the best treatment strategy for each patient.

References

1.	Cockerell OC, Johnson AL, Sander JW et al. Mortality of epilepsy: results from a prospective population-based study. *Lancet* 1994;344:918–21.
2.	Binnie CD, Chadwick D, Shorvon SD. Surgical Treatment for Epilepsy. ILAE Report British Branch of the International League against Epilepsy, 1991.
3.	Begley CE, Famulari M, Annegers JF et al. The cost of epilepsy in the United States: an estimate from population-based clinical and survey data. *Epilepsia* 2000;41:342–51.
4.	Hauser WA, Kurland LT. The epidemiology of epilepsy in Rochester, Minnesota 1935 through 1967. *Epilepsia* 1975;16:1–66.
5.	Nashef L, Fish DR, Sander JW et al. Incidence of sudden unexpected death in an adult outpatient cohort with epilepsy at a tertiary referral centre. *J Neurol Neurosurg Psychiatry* 1995;58:462–4.

6.   Nashef L, Fish DR, Garner S et al. Sudden death in epilepsy: a study of incidence in a young cohort with epilepsy and learning difficulty. *Epilepsia* 1995;36:1187–94.

7.   Shorvon SD, Laidlaw J, Richens A et al., editors. *A Textbook of Epilepsy*. 3rd edition. London: Churchill Livingstone, 1987.

8.   College of General Practitioners. A survey of epileptics in general practice. *BMJ* 1960;2:416–22.

9.   Office of Health Economics. *Epilepsy in Society*. London: Office of Health Economics, 1972.

10. Sillanpaa M. Children with epilepsy as adults: outcome after 30 years of follow-up. *Acta Paediatr Scand* 1990;79 (Suppl. 368):1–78.

11. Scambler G, Hopkins A. Social class, epileptic activity and disadvantage at work. *J Epidemiol Community Health* 1980;34:129–33.

12. Sander JW. Some aspects of prognosis in the epilepsies: a review. *Epilepsia* 1993;34:1007–16.

13. Sander JW, Hart YM, Johnson A et al. National General Practice Study of Epilepsy: newly diagnosed epileptic seizures in a general population. *Lancet* 1990;336:1267–71.

14. Placencia M, Suarez J, Crespo F et al. A large-scale study of epilepsy in Ecuador: methodological aspects. *Neuroepidemiology* 1992;11:74–84.

15. Gowers WR, editor. *Epilepsy and Other Chronic Convulsive Disorders*. London: Churchill Livingstone, 1881.

16. Rodin EA, editor. *The Prognosis of Patients with Epilepsy*. Springfield: Charles C Thomas, 1968.

17. Annegers JF, Hauser WA, Elveback LR. Remission of seizures and relapse in patients with epilepsy. *Epilepsia* 1979;20:729–37.

18. Goodridge DM, Shorvon SD. Epileptic seizures in a population of 6,000. I. Demography, diagnosis and classification, and role of the hospital services. *BMJ* 1983;287:641–4.

19. Pond D, Bidwell B, Stein L. A survey of 14 general practices. *Psychiatria Neurologia Neurochurugia* 1960;63:217–36.

20. Gudmundsson G. Epilepsy in Iceland. *Acta Neurol Scand* 1966;43 (Suppl. 25):1–124.

21. Cockerell OC, Eckel IE, Goodridge DM et al. Epilepsy in a population of 6,000 reexamined: secular trends in first attendance rates, prevalence and prognosis. *J Neurol Neurosurg Psychiatry* 1995;58:570–6.

22. Li LM, Fish DR, Sisodiya SM et al. High resolution MRI in adults with partial or secondary generalised epilepsy attending a tertiary referral unit. *J Neurol Neurosurg Psychiatry* 1995;59:384–7.

23. Binnie CD, Holder DS. Meinardi H, editors. *The Epilepsies*, Part I. Amsterdam: Elsevier, 1999:283–318.

24. Hajek M, Wieser HG, Khan N et al. Preoperative and postoperative glucose consumption in mesiobasal and lateral temporal lobe epilepsy. *Neurology* 1994;44:2125–32.

25. Henry TR, Sutherling WW, Engel J Jr et al. Interictal cerebral metabolism in partial epilepsies of neocortical origin. *Epilepsy Res* 1991;10:174–82.

26. Engel J Jr, Henry TR, Swartz BE et al., editors. *Epilepsy and the Functional Anatomy of the Frontal Lobe*. New York: Raven Press, 1995:223–38.

27. Engel J Jr, Kuhl DE, Phelps ME et al. Local cerebral metabolism during partial seizures. *Neurology* 1983;33:400–13.

28. Chugani HT, Rintahaka PJ, Shewmon DA. Ictal patterns of cerebral glucose utilization in children with epilepsy. *Epilepsia* 1994;35:813–22.

29. Prevett MC, Duncan JS, Jones T et al. Demonstration of thalamic activation during typical absence seizures using H2(15)O and PET. *Neurology* 1995;45:1396–402.

30. Koepp MJ, Richardson MP, Brooks DJ et al. Central benzodiazepine/gamma-aminobutyric acid A receptors in idiopathic generalized epilepsy: an [^{11}C]flumazenil positron emission tomography study. *Epilepsia* 1997;38:1089–97.

31. Prevett MC, Lammertsma AA, Brooks DJ et al. Benzodiazepine-GABA A receptors in idiopathic generalized epilepsy measured with [^{11}C]flumazenil and positron emission tomography. *Epilepsia* 1995;36:113–21.

32. Richardson MP, Koepp MJ, Brooks DJ et al. Cerebral activation in malformations of cortical development. *Brain* 1998;121:1295–304.

CHAPTER 2
Imaging techniques for epilepsy

Structural imaging techniques
Introduction
Up until the 1970s, the only techniques that allowed brain structure to be assessed were cerebral angiography and air encephalography. Cerebral angiography relies on deducing the presence of masses by patterns of shift in the blood vessels within the skull. With air encephalography, a lumbar puncture is performed and a small amount of air is injected into the spinal canal. The patient sits upright and air is allowed to float up and fill the cerebral ventricles. The ventricular outlines can be examined by x-ray to detect any deformities.

Both of these methods are indirect and only give a crude assessment of the presence or absence of an intracranial mass. Significant morbidities are also associated with both procedures: cerebral angiography carries a 1% risk of stroke and air encephalography causes severe headache in a significant proportion of patients. Since the advent of cross-sectional imaging techniques, angiography for indirect assessment and encephalography are now only of historical interest.

CT scans and MRI
Computed tomography (CT) scanning represented a major advance in structural imaging and allowed visualization of brain anatomy, as well as the localization of most intracranial masses. Some examples of anatomy and pathology on CT scans are shown in **Figure 2.1**. However, CT is insensitive to differences in brain tissue and so may fail to detect some of the structural lesions associated with epilepsy, such as gliomas and dysembryoplastic neuroepithelial tumors, as well as hippocampal sclerosis. CT scanning also necessitates a significant radiation dose and cannot be performed in different planes without moving the patient.

Magnetic resonance imaging (MRI) has allowed many of the limitations of CT scanning to be overcome. It provides better contrast resolution, which allows more accurate tissue definition and recognition of the lesions described above. Different types of resolution are defined in **Table 2.1**. Furthermore, MRI provides better spatial resolution. The combination of high spatial and contrast resolutions facilitates recognition of malformations of cortical development, which may underlie chronic epilepsy. MRI also does not involve a radiation dose and can be performed in any given plane without moving the patient. The major disadvantage of MRI over CT is that the patient has to lie still for longer.

Functional imaging techniques
Even with high-resolution structural imaging, only a small proportion of CT and MR scans demonstrate the cause of a patient's epilepsy. The remaining patients will either have a subtle structural cause that has not been detected or a nonstructural cause for their epilepsy. For this reason, newer techniques have been developed that

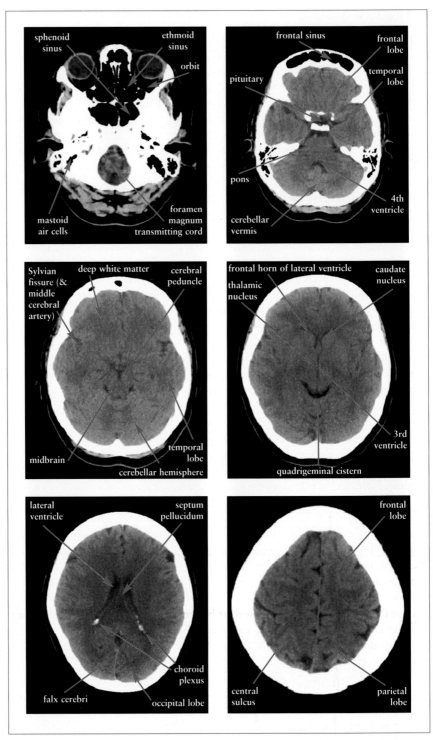

Figure 2.1. Examples of computed tomography brain scans. Axial sections through a normal brain.

Table 2.1. Definitions of the different types of resolution.

Spatial resolution	The ability of a scanning technique to demonstrate a small physical separation between two objects
Contrast resolution	The ability of a scanning technique to demonstrate a small difference in tissue characteristics between two objects
Temporal resolution	The ability of a scanning technique to demonstrate a small time difference between two events

image functional changes – e.g. changes in blood flow, concentrations of cellular constituents, or neurotransmitter binding – that are associated with epilepsy.

An overview of current functional imaging techniques is given in **Table 2.2**. The functional changes that underlie these techniques are discussed in more detail in Chapter 1 and the examples given are discussed in more detail in Chapter 3. The different imaging techniques are compared and contrasted in **Table 2.3**.

The first functional imaging study for epilepsy was published in 1988 [1]. The report described the imaging of brain perfusion using a phase mapping technique in a patient with continuous partial seizures. An area was identified in the frontal lobe that was abnormally perfused during a seizure (ictally) but which subsequently showed near normal perfusion after treatment.

Functional magnetic resonance imaging

Functional MRI (fMRI) encompasses a group of MR techniques that allow the physiological processes of neural activity to be measured in terms of local blood volume, flow, and oxygen saturation. Currently, fMRI allows imaging of brain function with spatial resolutions of 2–3 mm and temporal resolutions to within 1–2 seconds.

Cerebral blood volume-based techniques

In cerebral blood volume-based fMRI techniques, image contrast relies on the longstanding finding that neural activation is associated with an increase in local glucose metabolism and a subsequent increase in local cerebral blood flow [2]. The earliest fMRI methods compared the distribution of cerebral blood volume, with and without neural activation. Belliveau produced the first fMRI image of brain activity, which demonstrated increased blood flow to the primary visual cortex following visual stimulation [3].

Blood oxygenation level dependent imaging

In 1936, Linus Pauling described how the magnetic properties of hemoglobin (Hb) change with the state of oxygenation. In the deoxygenated form (deoxyhemoglobin), the Hb molecule has four of its six outer shell electrons unpaired. As a result, it acts in a paramagnetic fashion, i.e. it becomes magnetized in a strong magnetic field.

Table 2.2. Characteristics of the various imaging techniques currently available. BOLD: blood oxygenation level dependent; dwMRI: diffusion-weighted magnetic resonance imaging; fMRI: functional magnetic resonance imaging; MRS: magnetic resonance spectroscopy; PET: positron emission tomography; SPECT: single photon emission computed tomography.

(a) fMRI/BOLD imaging	
What can be measured?	Regions of increased blood flow in the brain
How is this process measured?	The MR signal of blood varies with its oxygenation. As blood flow increases to a region of the brain, its oxygenation also does. Hence, local blood flow can be deduced from changes in the MR signal
What are the applications of this technique in epilepsy?	Localization of the seizure focus, especially when the scan is electroencephalogram-triggered
	Mapping of the brain to localize functionally important regions before surgery

(b) PET imaging	
What can be measured?	Changes in glucose metabolism, and benzodiazepine, anticonvulsant, and opiate receptor distribution, which are all associated with epileptic foci
How is metabolism measured?	Radiopharmaceuticals – produced by the incorporation of radioisotopes into common brain metabolites – are injected into the patient and their uptake and metabolism are monitored, e.g. glucose metabolism is measured using ^{18}F-fluoro-deoxyglucose-PET
What are the applications of this technique in epilepsy?	Localization of the seizure focus

(c) SPECT imaging	
What can be measured?	Local cerebral blood flow and metabolism
How is metabolism measured?	Radiopharmaceuticals – the most common being ^{99}Tc^{m}-D,L-hexamethylpropyleneamineoxime – are injected into the patient and their uptake and metabolism are traced in 3 dimensions
What are the applications of this technique in epilepsy?	Comparison of interictal and ictal SPECT for identification of the epileptic focus

(d) MRS	
What can be measured?	Important chemical substances (bioconstituents) in the brain that are used in biological processes, such as lactate, choline, creatine, adenosine triphosphate, inorganic phosphate, and N-acetyl aspartate. It can also be used to measure the pH (using ratios of different phosphate molecules)
How are these bioconstituents measured?	The levels of various bioconstituents are determined using the frequency spectrum of a target nucleus (usually either ^{1}H or ^{32}P) that is contained within the bioconstituent being studied. MRS allows the measurement of a target nucleus within different bioconstituents
What are the applications of this technique in epilepsy?	MRS will give us a better knowledge of how these metabolites are linked to seizure activity. Certain bioconstituents are already known to be present in epileptic tissue and so measurements can be made to determine the focus of a patient's epilepsy

(e) dwMRI	
What can be measured?	Areas of disrupted macromolecular structure, e.g. areas of cerebral dysgenesis
	Continuous nerve tracts (since diffusion is easier along them)
How is it measured?	The apparent diffusion coefficient of water molecules is measured. The technique is based on the principle that diffusion will be easier along the axis of myelin fibers than across them. It is measured using a calculation derived from an MR scan.
What are the applications of this technique in epilepsy?	Identification of areas of cerebral dysgenesis that may be epileptogenic
	Localization of nerve tracts to assist surgical planning
	Detection of cell edema associated with status epilepticus (prolonged seizure)

Table 2.3. Comparison of functional imaging techniques used in epilepsy. fMRI: functional magnetic resonance imaging; MRS: magnetic resonance spectroscopy; PET: positron emission tomography; SPECT: single photon emission computed tomography.

Characteristic	fMRI	SPECT	PET	MRS
Spatial resolution	2–3 mm	10–15 mm	5–10 mm	~10 mm
Temporal resolution	Seconds	~1 minute	N/A	Hours
Quantification	Difficult	Difficult	Easy	Easy
Availability	Poor	Good	Poor	Poor
Ionizing radiation dose	Nil	5 mSv	10 mSv	Nil
Ictal/interictal availability	Interictal	Ictal and interictal	Interictal	Interictal
Anatomical detail	Yes	No	No	Yes

This magnetization causes an inhomogeneity and results in an overall decrease in MR signal. In its oxygenated form (oxyhemoglobin), an unpaired electron is transferred to the oxygen molecule, therefore eliminating the paramagnetic character and resulting in an increased MR signal [4]. During cerebral activation, physiological studies have shown that the extra oxygen flux supplied by the increased blood flow (typically in the order of 50%) exceeds metabolic requirements (oxygen consumption usually only rises by 5%). Therefore, in the active area, the ratio of oxygenated to deoxygenated blood is increased, as is the MR signal [5].

The fMRI community became aware that oxygenation level dependent differences in the magnetic properties of Hb could form the basis of cerebral fMRI contrast. This new technique was called blood oxygenation level dependent (BOLD) imaging. BOLD imaging rapidly became popular and it forms the basis of most fMRI work at present. It has considerable advantages over earlier methods because the contrast mechanism is endogenous and the administration of potentially toxic contrast media is not required. Images may be easily obtained using readily available conventional MR sequences. One limiting factor of fMRI for temporal resolution is that the blood flow response to cerebral activity does not begin until at least 2 seconds after stimulation, with a peak at about 10 seconds [6]. An example of auditory cortex identification using BOLD imaging is provided in **Figure 2.2**.

Design of fMRI experiments
The design of fMRI experiments to identify the cortical areas that serve a particular function can be problematic. The usual rationale is to subtract the activity in areas that are activated while doing a baseline task from the activity in areas that are activated while performing a particular task. This is relatively simple to determine for a motor task, for example, when the active portion is "finger tapping" and the baseline is "not finger tapping". However, with higher cortical functions, such as speech or cognitive tasks, careful thought must be given as to how the function

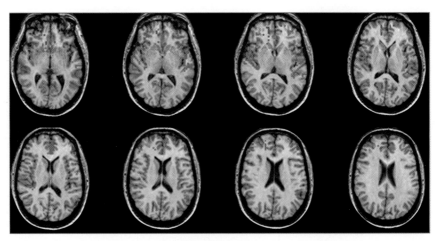

Figure 2.2. Blood oxygenation level dependent (BOLD) image showing auditory cortex identification. This figure is courtesy of Philips Medical.

under question can be isolated and stimulated reproducibly (see Chapter 4 for specific examples).

Experiments in healthy volunteers have revealed that the motor cortex (central gyrus) is activated by finger tapping, while the speech area is activated by a verbal fluency task. The occipital (visual) cortex is activated by the checkerboard and the sensory cortex (precentral gyrus) is activated by sensory stimulation. A task involving working memory is associated with activation of the prefrontal dorsolateral cortex (see **Figure 2.3**).

Postprocessing of fMRI data

Data from fMRI experiments are processed in two steps:

1. The MR signal data are analyzed to determine whether or not the task in question induces a change in signal corresponding to neural functioning.

2. Areas with increased activity are mapped onto a 3-dimensional MR image of a standardized brain and are warped to a predefined anatomical template to allow comparison between subjects, independent of brain size, shape, and orientation within the scanner. Brain areas shown to have increased activity may then be linked to the neural task in question.

The first step was originally carried out simply by subtracting the raw MR signal data for active and baseline tasks. However, it was found that noise fluctuations in the data sets were drowning out small activation signals, which were in the order of 2%–3%. Therefore, more sophisticated methods were developed based on statistical models, which determined the probability level of each area being activated.

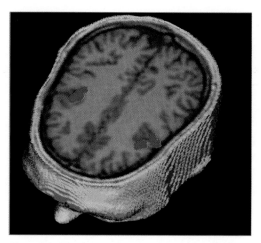

Figure 2.3. Blood oxygenation level dependent (BOLD) image showing activation of the prefrontal dorsolateral cortex; this indicates working memory. This figure is courtesy of Philips Medical.

Current approaches use Student's t statistic to calculate the probability that a given activation in a voxel (the smallest volume of tissue that can be physically resolved by the scanning sequence, about 1 mm³) has arisen by random noise fluctuation. Student's t statistic is determined by dividing the difference in the mean signal between the activated and baseline states by the pooled error (the latter is an estimate of the total variability in the data in both the inactivated and activated state). The neural activation task is repeated many times during the experiment, which helps reduce the statistical variability. In one of these current approaches, the statistical parametric map (SPM) program (see **Figure 2.4** for a simplified outline of the process) [7], each voxel is compared to every other voxel and Student's t statistic is determined. An image of the brain showing each voxel colored according to its t statistic is the SPM. A threshold is set for lighting up a voxel, e.g. a t statistic of greater than 5 (which indicates that the probability of a difference in a voxel's signal arising by chance is less than 1 in 10^5, i.e. 0.001%). In this way, a probabilistic activation map is obtained showing areas of observed increased activation that are unlikely to be due to chance alone.

An advantage of fMRI over other functional imaging modalities, such as positron emission tomography (PET), is that the image can be acquired in the same session as a high-quality structural MR scan. The structural and functional images are usually grossly compatible on a voxel-by-voxel basis (since movement between the two scans will be minimal), although some geometric distortion can occur because of varying artifacts in the different MR sequences used for each acquisition. Various postprocessing computer routines have been developed to correct for this.

The structural MR scan can be analyzed (e.g. using programs produced by the Montreal Neurological Institute) to determine the degree of warping required to normalize the subject's brain to a standardized brain template. This warping can then be applied to the functional data so that an image of neurofunctional activation on a standardized brain can be obtained, which can form a basis for comparison between different subjects and different neural activation tasks.

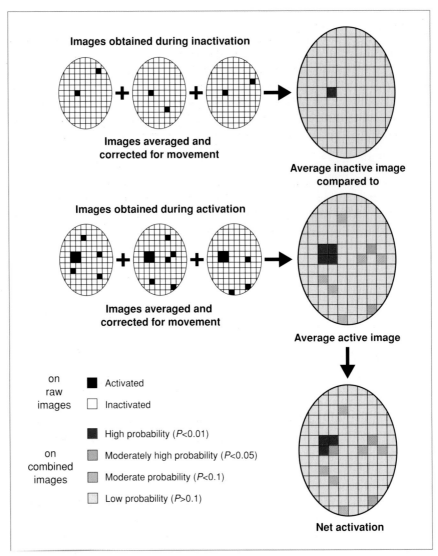

Figure 2.4. A simplified example of the statistical parametric map (SPM) program. A series of images during "inactivation" or "nonactivation" are combined to form an average inactive image. Similarly, an average active image is obtained from the combination of images obtained during activation. The inactive image is compared to the active image and, using a complex series of statistical calculations, a probabilistic map is generated in which each voxel is assigned a probability that it has been activated.

Methodological problems with fMRI
Difficulties in defining the eloquent cortex
When setting up a cerebral activation task, or series of tasks, one disadvantage of fMRI is that only information about a single specific neural function can be obtained from each experiment. It has been shown that even the processing of single words induces activation of parallel sensory-specific, phonological, articulatory, and semantic coding areas [8]. Several approaches have been proposed to overcome these problems.

Subtraction

The most widely used approach is subtraction. In this method, two tasks are devised that are quite similar, differing only in the neural activation for which imaging is required. For example, activation during reading words aloud and activation while reading words silently, with the difference between the two tasks being taken to represent motor speech activity. The subtraction method does have some weaknesses, most notably the assumption that complex neural tasks can be parcellated and that subtraction of part of a task will not affect the pathway of neural activation.

Attentional modulation

With this technique, almost all the experimental conditions are identical, except the instructions given to the patient. These instructions specify concentrating on a particular aspect for one part of the experiment and no particular aspect for the other part of the experiment. The difference in activations is taken to represent the value that results from focusing on the specific neural task. For example, subjects might be asked to look at a series of moving shapes and then to pay attention to their color and perhaps their motion. This experimental design assumes that the neural processing involved in using a skill, such as shape perception, unconsciously is much less than the neural processing when using the skill consciously – the subtracted activation largely represents the neural task.

Stimulus modulation

In this technique, the neural task for which the processing correlate is required is varied in terms of intensity or frequency. The processed data are then examined to determine whether or not the neural activity variation correlates with stimulus variation. This method of experimental design can only be performed if a particular neural process can be modulated in a stepwise fashion and if modulation is proportional to stimulation.

fMRI in children

Younger children may not be able to cooperate with some of the functional paradigms used. Indeed, they may not be able to endure any form of imaging without sedation or general anesthetic. The situation may improve as alternate paradigms are developed that prove to be sensitive, specific, and reproducible. The imaging methods involving ionizing radiation generally require only basic patient cooperation. However, there is a natural reluctance to use them in children because of concerns about cancer induction – although the risks have been shown to be extremely small [10].

fMRI in epilepsy

Preoperative mapping of functionally important cortex

Until recently, the only available method to predict whether a patient was going to suffer an unacceptable neurological deficit from removal or ablation of epileptogenic tissue was to perform a craniotomy, implant subdural electrodes, and use functional mapping studies to determine the exact location of the motor area, speech area, and so on. This procedure is either performed separately before the operation or at the beginning of the operation. In the latter case, the patient requires a short-acting

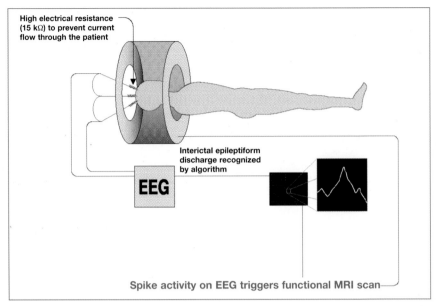

High electrical resistance
(15 kΩ) to prevent current
flow through the patient

Interictal epileptiform
discharge recognized
by algorithm

EEG

Spike activity on EEG triggers functional MRI scan

Figure 2.5. Illustration of electroencephalography (EEG) triggered magnetic resonance imaging (MRI). The patient's EEG is continuously monitored and when a series of interictal epileptiform discharges (IED) occurs, the functional scan is triggered to demonstrate increased activity in the irritative area generating IEDs.

general anesthetic and is awakened for functional testing after the craniotomy has been performed.

Direct intracranial stimulation has several associated problems when compared with fMRI:

- It is invasive.
- Only a small area of cortex can be exposed and tested from a craniotomy.
- Testing is limited by time and patient comfort.
- Repeated electrical stimulation near the seizure focus can itself induce seizures, which can make accurate mapping difficult and can obscure the extent of the eloquent cortex because of electrical spread.

Direct cortical stimulation does have some advantages over functional mapping. Most importantly, a cortical area that on stimulation is found to be related to a neurological function will certainly be involved primarily in the execution of that task, whereas, in an fMRI experiment, other cerebral areas may be activated that are not directly involved but are related to the neurological task (see Chapter 4).

EEG triggering

Electroencephalogram (EEG) triggering (see **Figure 2.5**) is a technique that has recently been developed to allow fMRI to be performed during interictal epileptiform discharges (IEDs) in the irritative zone. IEDs are electrical changes that can be detected on the EEG and are thought to arise from the region of cortex that generates the epileptic seizures. More IEDs are produced before a seizure and their appearance

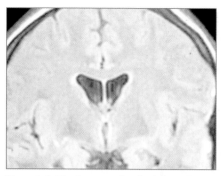

Figure 2.6. Blood oxygenation level dependent (BOLD) image demonstrating electroencephalography (EEG) triggering.

is considered to reflect low-grade epileptic activity that has not reached the threshold for a clinically apparent seizure.

There are considerable practical advantages in being able to trigger based on IEDs:

- The patient does not have to wait until he or she has a seizure (seizures may be occasional and unpredictable).
- The patient does not have to endure the discomfort and safety hazards of a seizure in the scanner.

Defining the irritative zone – which tends to correlate well with the epileptogenic lesion, even if it is not obvious on a structural MR scan – is potentially more valuable than defining the epileptogenic or symptomogenic zones, which are excited later during ictus and may not correlate well with the underlying lesion. Thus, EEG triggering may prove to be particularly useful in the presurgical setting to define the area of cortex that can beneficially be resected.

Prior to the development of this technique, a number of technical and safety issues had to be overcome. Technical issues include EEG artifacts generated by high and varying magnetic fields in the scanner. These obscure fine detail and require the use of specially developed filter algorithms. Safety issues include the risk of an electromotive force being generated in the EEG electrodes and attached wires due to the rapidly changing magnetic field. To avoid this, the current in the electrodes is limited by the use of large resistors (15,000 Ohms). Reproducibility is improved by averaging out functional data from up to 60 IEDs [9]. An example of an early sequence (the spatial resolution has since been improved) demonstrating BOLD activation from EEG triggering is shown in **Figure 2.6.**

Single photon emission computed tomography

Single photon emission computed tomography (SPECT) imaging appears to be a particularly promising technique and has already been widely taken up by various groups for imaging ictal foci. It is a refinement of ordinary gamma camera imaging in which the uptake and distribution of a gamma-ray emitting-radiopharmaceutical are followed in planar images. Images are reconstructed to display a series of 2-dimensional slices at different levels through the subject. Thus, the distribution of the radiotracer in 3 dimensions can be pinpointed. However, for technical reasons, the spatial resolution achieved (10–15 mm) is not as good as with a conventional gamma camera.

The radiopharmaceutical consists of a radioactive atom chemically tagged to a natural substance/pharmaceutical. The radioisotope most commonly used is technetium-99m ($^{99}Tc^m$), a radioactive element produced by the decay of molybdenum-99. It is a man-made radioisotope that is produced in a nuclear reactor. $^{99}Tc^m$ has many ideal properties as a radionuclide, as explained in **Table 2.4.**

Table 2.4. Ideal properties of technetium ($^{99}Tc^m$) as a radionuclide.

1. Tc can be produced in a desk-mounted generator unit containing a lead-shielded column of molybdenum-99 (^{99}Mo). ^{99}Mo decays to $^{99}Tc^m$ with a half-life of 67 hours. $^{99}Tc^m$ itself decays to ^{99}Tc with a half-life of 6 hours. The $^{99}Tc^m$ is extracted every 24 hours by washing though a column with sterile saline. This 24-hour interval is practical because it allows the $^{99}Tc^m$ to build up on a daily basis to a maximum equilibrium level (since it is being constantly produced but is also constantly decaying). After a week, the ^{99}Mo is largely exhausted and the generator is returned to the manufacturer.

2. When $^{99}Tc^m$ decays to ^{99}Tc, gamma photons are emitted, predominantly with an energy of 140 keV. The monoenergetic nature of the emission is advantageous, since it allows scattered photons of lower energy, which would blur the image, to be filtered out. This energy (140 keV) is high enough to exit the patient but low enough to be easily collimated and measured. Fortunately no α or β radiation is emitted, since these radiations would not contribute to the patient's image and would only deposit an extra radiation dose in the patient.

3. As ^{99}Tc itself decays very slowly, with a half-life of 213,000 years, it does not contribute to the image.

$^{99}Tc^m$ can be linked to various pharmaceuticals, the most common being D,L-hexamethylpropyleneamineoxime (HMPAO). HMPAO is a lipophilic complex, which crosses the blood–brain barrier and localizes in tissues according to the local cerebral blood flow. It is highly extracted on first pass with very little redistribution. Most (80%–90%) of the compound remains where it was first taken up 24 hours after it was administered.

The SPECT scan

Since the SPECT image obtained is dependent on cerebral blood flow, conditions under which the scan is performed are standardized as much as possible. The scan is performed in a quiet room with no visual or aural distractions. The patient has an intravenous cannula placed before the scan is carried out. Up to 500 MBq of radiopharmaceutical (usually $^{99}Tc^m$–HMPAO) are injected and scanning can be performed any time from 5 minutes to 24 hours later.

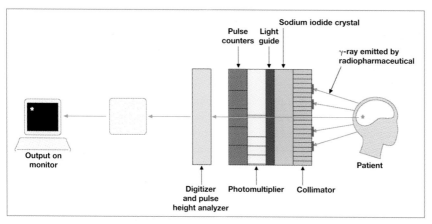

Figure 2.7. Diagram showing the mechanism of action of the gamma camera. Gamma rays emitted by brain areas are first collimated to eliminate any rays that are not passing perpendicular to the gamma camera (these rays would worsen the image quality). Within the sodium iodide crystal, gamma rays are converted to photons of light, are multiplied by the photomultiplier, and are finally converted into electrical pulses. These pulses are counted, analyzed, and digitized for graphical display on a computer screen.

Ictal SPECT is a modification of the technique. The patient has an intravenous cannula placed for up to 48 hours with close monitoring. When he or she is about to have a seizure (the patient may either warn the staff of a recognizable aura or an observer may notice), the radiopharmaceutical is injected by a nurse or doctor. This sequence of events requires trained staff who are able to monitor the patient closely and administer the injection safely. Suitable equipment should be available to document the seizure on video and, if possible, using an EEG. The injected $^{99}Tc^m$–HMPAO is rapidly fixed for 12–24 hours in the brain, giving a "snapshot" of the ictal metabolic activity.

A gamma camera is used to image the gamma ray emission from the patient (see **Figure 2.7**). This contains a solid sodium iodide crystal measuring about 50 cm in diameter with a thickness of 9–12 mm. The crystal absorbs about 90% of the gamma rays that pass through it and converts each gamma photon into approximately 5,000 light photons that travel in all directions. About 4,000 of these photons emerge from the back surface of the crystal, where the light output is passed through an array of tightly packed photomultiplier tubes. The light photons are converted and multiplied to generate electrical pulses.

The crystal is well shielded to prevent extraneous radiation, e.g. cosmic rays, which may cause interference. To ensure that each position of the electrical pulses generated by the gamma camera corresponds to a particular point within the patient, a collimator (a lead plate about 40 cm in diameter with a thickness of 2.5 cm) is placed in front of the crystal. Up to 20,000 circular hexagonal holes are drilled through the thickness of the plate. The collimator filters out any gamma rays that are not travelling at 90° to it (in practice, about 95% of the radiation incident on the collimator is filtered out).

In straightforward planar gamma camera imaging, the camera is static. In SPECT imaging, the gamma camera rotates in a circle around the patient and a tomographic image is obtained using a reconstruction technique [4]. The SPECT camera stops every 6° for 20–30 seconds, with 60 views being obtained from a 360° rotation in about 30 minutes. If the patient moves during the scan, considerable spatial inaccuracy is introduced into the reconstruction algorithm. The maximum practical scan duration is approximately 30 minutes, since most people are unable to stay still for longer than this. Because of collimation (which filters out a large proportion of the photons) and because the camera can only spend a few seconds on each "view" of the patient, relatively few counts are obtained during the SPECT scan compared with the number obtained during a PET scan. The low number of photons used to form the image increases the relative contribution of random variation (quantum noise). This increases the noise in the image and degrades the spatial resolution. The advantages and limitations of SPECT are provided in **Table 2.5.**

Table 2.5. Advantages and limitations of SPECT.

Advantages	Limitations
Less expensive than PET because of the longer half-life of tracers	Involves the use of intravenous radiolabeled substances
Unlike PET, a nearby cyclotron unit is not needed; therefore, it is a more widely available technique	The spatial resolution of SPECT (8–10 mm) is not as good as that of PET – precise localization is not possible
An expanding range of radiotracer compounds with long half-life values enhances the range of SPECT applications	
State-of-the-art cameras and collimators offer improved spatial resolution	

Ictal and interictal SPECT studies in a patient with hippocampal sclerosis revealed by MRI are illustrated in **Figure 2.8.** These studies show that the left temporal lobe is hypometabolic interictally and hypermetabolic ictally. Therefore, functional evidence can be added to structural findings.

Radiation dosimetry
The whole body radiation dose for a $^{99}Tc^m$ HMPAO SPECT study is 5 mSv.

SISCOM coregistration
Relating seizure neurophysiology to anatomy – e.g. for presurgical planning – is difficult. Interictal and ictal SPECT images and MR images cannot easily be compared side-by-side because slice locations and orientations will vary. Therefore, the technique of subtraction SPECT with coregistration mapping (SISCOM) has been developed. Using SISCOM, SPECT images are normalized, realigned, subtracted from each other (generating a map of blood flow changes), and

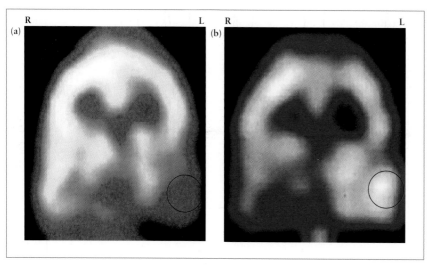

Figure 2.8. Hippocampal sclerosis shown by single photon emission computed tomography. The interictal study (a) shows decreased metabolism in the left temporal lobe and the ictal study (b) shows increased metabolism in a similar area. L: left; R: right.

coregistered onto a high-resolution MR scan. As a result, the anatomical regions involved in the scan can be confidently identified [11]. SISCOM improves the sensitivity and reproducibility of SPECT scans.

Positron emission tomography

PET has been rapidly endorsed by the research community, as it offers the most comprehensive noninvasive way to look at biologically active metabolites *in vivo*. PET uses positron-emitting radioisotopes, typically incorporated into labeled versions of common metabolites, to measure changes in cerebral blood flow and energy metabolism caused by neuronal activity. PET was developed in the late 1970s, with the first reported use in 1977 [12]. The first symposium on applications of PET was in 1978 [13]. Almost from the outset it was realized that this technique could be used to map cerebral blood flow: in 1980, Frackowiak reported normal values for the human brain [14].

Radioisotopes used in PET are typically produced by the bombardment of stable isotopes with positively charged particles, such as protons or deuterium nuclei. Because of the short half-lives of the radioisotopes produced, they must be incorporated immediately into the desired compounds. Therefore, a nearby cyclotron and radiochemical laboratory are required, rendering PET a relatively laborious and expensive technique. PET radiopharmaceuticals can only provide meaningful metabolic information of steady-state conditions and this factor, along with their short half-life, renders them unsuitable for ictal scanning (unless PET scanning can be performed in a patient with continuous focal epilepsy).

Because of the short half-life of PET radiopharmaceuticals (with the exception of ^{18}F-fluoro-deoxyglucose [FDG]), the activity from a particular area of uptake may fall off significantly during the scan. A computer algorithm needs to be applied to correct for this. This algorithm works best when the PET radiopharmaceutical is delivered as a single bolus to the areas of interest, necessitating intra-arterial delivery via an arterial line. Currently available PET radioisotopes, their half-lives, and methods of production are listed in **Table 2.6.**

Table 2.6. Common PET radioisotopes.

Radioisotope	Produced by bombardment of	Bombarding particle	Half-life (minutes)
^{11}C	^{14}N	Proton	20
^{13}N	^{12}C	Deuterium nucleus	10
^{15}O	^{14}N	Deuterium nucleus	2
^{18}F	^{20}Ne or ^{18}O or proton	Deuterium nucleus	110

The ability to radiolabel atoms that are common constituents of most biological compounds has allowed the development of a series of biological radiopharmaceuticals that can be used to image many metabolic functions (see **Table 2.7**).

Table 2.7. Common PET radiopharmaceuticals.

Radiopharmaceutical	Metabolic function imaged
^{18}F-fluoro-deoxyglucose	Glucose metabolism
^{18}O-O_2	Oxygen metabolism
^{15}O-H_2O	Cerebral blood flow
^{11}C-flumazenil	Benzodiazepine receptor distribution
^{11}C-carfentanil	Opiate receptor distribution
^{11}C-phenytoin	Anticonvulsant distribution
^{11}C-valproate	Anticonvulsant distribution

PET – the physics

Since positron emitters are created by the bombardment of neutral atoms with positively charged particles, they are proton-rich. The radioisotopes seek to lose excess positive charge by the emission of a positively charged electron, or positron, which is produced by the breakdown of a proton into a neutron plus a positron. The positron is emitted by the nucleus and travels for a very short path (usually between 2–5 mm) before colliding with an electron in surrounding tissue. When a positron collides with an electron, both particles are annihilated with the conversion of mass into energy. The energy is released in the form of two photons of fixed energy (511 keV) travelling at 180° to each other. The photons are detected by a positron

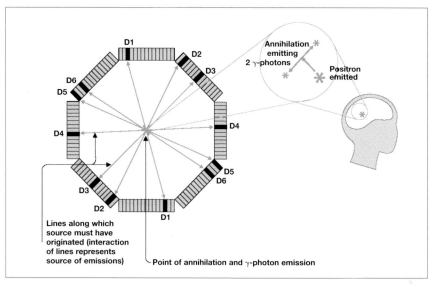

Figure 2.9. Diagrammatic representation of PET. Positrons emitted by a radiopharmaceutical in active brain areas are almost immediately annihilated with the production of two photons traveling at 180° to each other, which are detected by detector pair D1. Further positrons emitted are detected by pairs D2–D6. By calculating the intersection of lines joining the detector pairs, the location of the source can be calculated and the activated brain area can be demonstrated.

camera (which uses photomultiplier tubes as in SPECT imaging), which localizes and quantifies the positron emitter. However, unlike SPECT, the photodetecting array is arranged in a ring or hexagon around the patient. The most commonly used photodetector is bismuth germinate (although some more modern materials are becoming more widely used).

A circuit is set up (see **Figure 2.9**) with a signal only being registered if detectors on opposite sides of the body each register a blip simultaneously. Therefore, if an event is registered, the positron emitter must have been somewhere along a line connecting the two detectors. As the emitter continues to emit, successive events are registered in different pairs of detectors. Lines drawn from each pair of detectors registering an event will intersect at the location of the positron emitter. This method allows reliable identification of the position of the positron emitter without collimation (unlike SPECT). The positron camera array consists of many detectors, so a 2-dimensional picture of the positron emission can be built up by filtered back projection (as described for SPECT).

Some resolution limitations are inherent in PET. Firstly, because the positrons travel for a short distance before annihilation, resolution can never be less than to a few millimeters. Secondly, the electron and positron are not completely at rest when annihilation occurs. This introduces a slight change to the angle between the two emitted photons resulting in them not being exactly 180° to each other, and causes some more spatial resolution error. Other limitations arise from errors introduced by detectors and postprocessing.

Coregistration may be performed by reorientating, normalizing, and superimposing the image onto a high-resolution MR scan in a similar way to that described for SPECT. As PET is sensitive to metabolic changes, continuous scalp EEG monitoring is usually performed before and after administration of the radiopharmaceutical to determine the state of wakefulness, the frequency of interictal discharges, and the occurrence of subclinical (electrographic) seizures. Advantages and limitations of PET are provided in **Table 2.8**.

Table 2.8. Advantages and limitations of PET.

Advantages	Limitations
Facilitates the assessment of receptor distribution in the brain	PET is expensive and is unlikely to be available for routine clinical use
Measurement of cerebral blood flow during neuropsychological testing allows mapping of regions of cerebral activation during cognitive or motor tasks	A local radiochemistry department is required for the production of radiotracer substances, since the half-life of these compounds is short
PET cerebral glucose metabolism can reflect resting brain activity or metabolism during a cognitive task	The radiation dose limits repeated scanning. Using lower doses of radiotracer minimizes this problem but prolongs the scanning time
Improved anatomic localization of activity is possible by overlaying PET scan information onto MR images	Low spatial and temporal resolutions compared with fMRI

Radiation dosimetry

The typical activities that are used are 350–700 MBq for ^{11}C-ligands and 200–400 MBq for ^{18}F-ligands, giving a total radiation dose of 5–10 mSv per study.

Magnetic resonance spectroscopy

Magnetic resonance spectroscopy (MRS) allows the *in vivo* assessment of molecules involved in a variety of neural processes, e.g. components of cell membranes, neurotransmitters, and compounds involved in energy usage. It is performed in an extended MR scanning session, taking longer than a conventional structural MR scan.

MRI depends upon the generation of a magnetic field within which certain nuclei, including ^{1}H, ^{13}C, and ^{31}P, will display the quantum mechanical property of "spin". These nuclei can be considered to be small magnetic dipoles. Nuclei are excited by an electromagnetic pulse, called the RF pulse. The frequency is set so that nuclei (usually hydrogen, i.e. protons) in the target volume will resonate optimally, or precess. As the nuclei precess they emit tiny magnetic signals that are received by a detecting coil and analyzed as a frequency spectrum (see **Figure 2.10**).

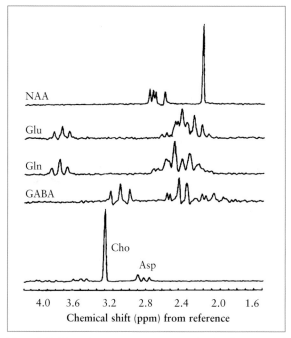

Figure 2.10. Magnetic resonance spectroscopy showing the position of metabolites detected by ^{1}H (proton) spectroscopy, as determined by their chemical shift pattern. Asp: aspartate; Cho: choline; GABA: gamma-aminobutyric acid; Gln: glutamine; Glu: glutamate; NAA: N-acetyl aspartate.

The target volume may be defined using two different methods. With the first method – the single voxel technique – a single volume of interest is defined and examined. This technique allows sampling of only a small area of brain (typically approximately 8 mL for ^{1}H and 60–100 mL for ^{31}P spectroscopy); therefore, prior knowledge of the area that is likely to be abnormal is required.

The second method is chemical shift imaging (CSI), also known as magnetic resonance spectroscopy imaging (MRSI). With this technique a large region of tissue is excited and the spectroscopic signals from different voxels are spatially encoded using phase-encoded gradients. This allows smaller voxels to be defined and studied (typically 1–2 mL for ^{1}H and 25 mL for ^{31}P spectroscopy). This technique is the preferred method, although it does pose greater technical challenges.

With MRS, the frequency spectrum for the target nucleus, e.g. ^{1}H or ^{31}P, is closely analyzed. The same nuclei within different chemical compounds will resonate at slightly different frequencies. This frequency will depend on the chemical surroundings, as the magnetic environment is affected by the electron cloud of nearby atoms (this phenomenon is known as "chemical shift artifact"). One common compound in which the nucleus in question appears is denoted the "reference compound". The change in resonant frequency from that of the nucleus in the reference compound is known as the "chemical shift" (this is measured as a proportion of the resonant frequency of the reference compound).

Chemical shifts are in the order of parts per million (ppm) and have been characterized for different molecules containing the nucleus being studied. Thus, for ^{31}P, the biologically important forms that are usually studied are:

- phosphocreatine (PCr)
- adenosine triphosphate (ATP)
- phosphomonoesters, including phosphorylcholine and phosphorylethanolamine
- phosphodiesters, including glycerolphosphorylcholine and glycerolphosphorylethanolamine
- inorganic phosphate (Pi)

Studying these molecules allows brain energy metabolism to be analyzed. The PCr/ATP ratio is a measure of metabolic status, since cerebral ATP is only usually exhausted under conditions of extreme stress. ^{31}P MRS also allows measurement of the intracellular pH. At physiological levels the Pi signal is an average of two contributing species, HPO_4^{2-} and $H_2PO_4^-$. The equilibrium between these two molecules reflects the intracellular pH.

^{31}P was the first nucleus to be used for brain MRS but its use is limited because of the poor signal to noise ratio obtained. However, the compounds detected using ^{31}P MRS are reasonably well separated with an overall range of about 30 ppm as opposed to ^{1}H MRS in which the range is about 10 ppm. Therefore, the minimal sample volumes using ^{31}P MRS are relatively large compared with the volumes used for ^{1}H MRS. ^{1}H MRS is far more sensitive, with signal to noise ratios around 14 times those of ^{31}P MRS.

^{1}H MRS allows the measurement of peaks in N-acetyl aspartate (NAA), creatine (Cr) containing compounds (principally Cr and PCr), and choline (Cho) containing compounds. In the brain, NAA is primarily located within neurons, whereas Cr, PCr, and Cho containing compounds are usually found in a wider range of cell types; higher concentrations are detected in oligodendrocytes and astrocytes than in neurons.

Lactate can also be measured using more advanced spectral editing techniques. Lactate is a marker of anaerobic glycolysis, a process that is thought to occur during ictus. Since this process is only evident under conditions of metabolic stress, it may prove to be more specific for identifying epileptic foci than ^{18}F-FDG PET, which relies on glucose to image both aerobic, i.e. physiological, and anaerobic metabolism.

Detection of gamma-aminobutyric acid (GABA) using ^{1}H MRS is technically difficult because its resonance signal overlaps with that of NAA and Cr and its concentration is also relatively low in the brain. However, detection has recently become possible using complex spectral editing techniques. These recent advances have also made it possible to measure other neurotransmitters, such as glutamate, glutamine, and inositol (the last is used as a measure of glial cell integrity). Advantages and limitations of MRS are provided in **Table 2.9**.

Table 2.9. Advantages and limitations of MRS.

Advantages	Limitations
Offers a relatively sophisticated method of assessing brain metabolism	Suffers from a relative lack of sensitivity – some metabolites that are present in low concentrations are not detectable
Potential aid in early diagnosis and subsequent monitoring of illness	
Allows determination of pharmaco-kinetic and also pharmacodynamic properties of neurological and psychiatric drugs	Transient biochemical changes are difficult to detect
	Poor resolution properties make it difficult to distinguish between biochemically similar compounds

Technical difficulties associated with MRS

MRS is technically challenging for a number of reasons:

- MRSI relies on frequency shifts that are used in structural MR scans for point localization within the area being studied; therefore, a different method of point localization must be used, prolonging the scan time.
- Because the frequency shifts are only in the order of ppm, the magnetic field must be uniform to within 1 ppm – this is especially true for MRSI.
- The predominant resonant signal returned from biological tissue arises from water protons: with ^{31}P MRS this predominating signal needs to be filtered out (especially for MRSI); ^{1}H MRS is a more sensitive technique because of a greater signal to noise ratio.
- High-specification MR equipment is required, with high-field magnets of 2 tesla or more to overcome these problems.
- MRSI is prone to leakage of signal from fat into nearby voxels. This can particularly cause problems when assessing the anterior temporal lobe structures, such as hippocampi.

MRS in epilepsy patients

NAA, creatine, and choline

A reduction in the NAA/(Cr+Cho) ratio has been observed in the affected lobe of patients with epilepsy arising from one cerebral lobe when compared with healthy subjects. In one study, the decrease in NAA was 22%, the increase in Cr was 15%, and the increase in Cho was 25% [15]. These findings indicate neuronal dysfunction or loss in the affected area, possibly associated with some gliosis. An example of these changes in a patient with unilateral focal epilepsy is provided in **Figure 2.11**.

Lactate

A postictal increase in lactate has been demonstrated in patients with focal epilepsy [16]. In the temporal lobe of patients with temporal lobe epilepsy, a postictal focal increase and a unilateral increase in lactate have been demonstrated. This is in contrast to the finding that the NAA/(Cr+Cho) ratio decreases bilaterally, indicating that lactate may be used as a direct measure of epileptic activity.

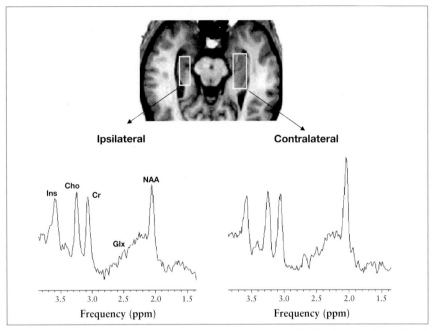

Ipsilateral   Contralateral

Figure 2.11. Magnetic resonance spectroscopy image showing unilateral focal epilepsy. In the unaffected (contralateral) side of the brain there is a normal ratio of N-acetyl aspartate (NAA) to the sum of choline (Cho) and creatine (Cr). In the affected (ipsilateral) side of the brain there is a decreased concentration of NAA relative to the sum of Cho and Cr. This indicates the breakdown of neuronal structure, which is consistent with gliosis. Glx: glutamine + glutamate; Ins: inositol. This figure is courtesy of Dr M McLean, National Society of Epilepsy.

GABA

There is a correlation between the control of seizures and brain GABA levels [17]. Drug-induced variations in the levels of brain GABA and its metabolites, homocarnosine and 2-pyrrolidinone, have also been observed during treatment with anticonvulsants, such as topiramate, vigabatrin, and gabapentin.

Diffusion-weighted magnetic resonance imaging

Diffusion-weighted magnetic resonance imaging (dwMRI) is an MRI approach that was developed in the 1980s. The technique measures changes in the apparent diffusion coefficient (ADC) of water in brain regions. It can be used to detect very early changes in cell edema after an acute cerebral infarct and may be useful in epilepsy for defining the anatomy of the neural tracts and detecting early cell edema after the epileptic ictus.

The technique of dwMRI takes advantage of the variable diffusion of water molecules in tissue. Molecules move in a random pattern when they are excited by thermal energy. This constant movement is called Brownian motion. In brain tissue this diffusion is not entirely random because of tissue structure and the interaction of water molecules with other macromolecules. During a typical MR observation time of 40 ms, molecules in pure water at room temperature travel approximately 10–30 μm, about twice the distance that water travels in body tissue. Therefore, the

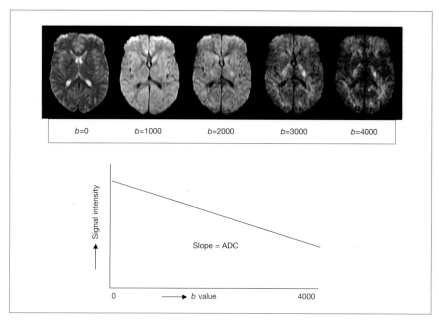

Figure 2.12. An example of a normal brain with a gradually increasing *b* value. In practice, a series of diffusion images are taken with varying *b* values and the apparent diffusion coefficient (ADC) is calculated from a complex plot that consists of the signals from brain tissues against *b*. The *b* value shows the relative contribution of the diffusion weighting to the already T2 weighted image, from *b*=0 where there is no contribution to *b*=4000 where the image is almost completely diffusion weighted (note that the high T2 signal of cerebrospinal fluid is gradually lost). This figure is courtesy of Philips Medical.

movement of water molecules in the brain is called "apparent diffusion". Water proton displacement is often expressed as the ADC, which mathematically is:

$$ADC = L^2 / (2\Delta T)$$
Where L is the average displacement in one direction during a time interval ΔT.

The ADC is decreased under circumstances where protons are slowed (but not completely stopped) in their random motion by cell membranes. The movement of water protons along myelin fibers will be greater along a certain axis, i.e. the movement along the fibers will be easier than the movement across them. Consequently, the diffusion of the proton may be described as anisotropic, i.e. not equal in all directions. (ADC and anisotropy maps can be used to express findings from diffusion studies.)

Clinical studies from about 1992 onwards showed that the ADC was regionally decreased in areas of acute cerebral infarct. The actual mechanism for this is still not entirely clear but it is thought to reflect the influx of relatively fast diffusing extracellular water into the more restricted intracellular environment. Therefore, as the neural cells swell with cytoxic edema, the frequency and magnitude of diffusion decreases. The reduced water ADC appears as an area of high signal on a dwMRI scan. During prolonged membrane depolarization, as occurs in status epilepticus, there is marked cell edema, which can be visualized by diffusion-weighted imaging.

Technical considerations with dwMRI

Different MR sequences are now available for dwMRI, each of which has several associated advantages and disadvantages. With most sequences, the combination of scan parameters is summarized by the b value, which can vary from zero (where there is an MR image with mainly T2 weighting but no diffusion weighting) up to a typical value of 600–800 seconds/mm² (where the image is mainly diffusion weighted). An example of a normal brain with a gradually increasing b value is provided in **Figure 2.12**.

Since contrast is generated by measuring small degrees of movement during dwMRI, the greatest problems arise from patient motion. This includes both voluntary and involuntary head movements, respiratory motion, and cardiac pulsation of the brain and cerebrospinal fluid. The effect of these movements can be reduced by spin echo-based imaging using a "navigator" sequence, which corrects misregistration of phase encoding steps. One disadvantage of this system is that it takes a relatively long time (up to 10 minutes) to acquire an image.

An alternative approach is to use a high-speed sequence called echo planar imaging or EPI. The disadvantage of this approach is that it uses gradient echoes, making it sensitive to susceptibility artifact, which appears at interfaces of tissues with different magnetic susceptibilities.

References

1. Fish DR, Brooks DJ, Young IR et al. Use of magnetic resonance imaging to identify changes in cerebral blood flow in epilepsia partialis continua. *Magn Reson Med* 1988;8:238–40.
2. Roy CS, Sherrington CS. On the regulation of the blood supply of the brain. *J Physiol* (London) 1890;11:85–108.
3. Belliveau JW, Kennedy DN Jr, McKinstry RC et al. Functional mapping of the human visual cortex by magnetic resonance. *Science* 1991;254:716–9.
4. Farr RF, Allisy-Roberts PJ. *Physics for Medical Imaging*. London: WB Saunders, 1998.
5. Fox PT, Raichle ME, Mintun MA et al. Nonoxidative glucose consumption during focal physiologic neural activity. *Science* 1988;241:462–4.
6. Kwong KK, Belliveau JW, Chesler DA et al. Dynamic magnetic resonance imaging of human brain activity during primary sensory stimulation. *Proc Natl Acad Sci USA* 1992;89:5675–9.
7. The Wellcome Department of Cognitive Neurology. Statistical Parametric Mapping. Available at: URL: http//www.fil.ion.ucl.ac.uk/spm/ Accessed on May 21, 2003.
8. Shorvon SD, Laidlaw J, Richens A et al, editors. *A Textbook of Epilepsy*. 3rd edition. London: Churchill Livingstone, 1987.
9. Krakow K, Woermann FG, Symms MR et al. EEG-triggered functional MRI of interictal epileptiform activity in patients with partial seizures. *Brain* 1999;122:1679–88.
10. Shulkin BL. PET application in pediatrics. *QJ Nucl Med* 1997;41:281–91.
11. Brinkmann BH, O'Brien TJ, Mullan BP et al. Subtraction ictal SPECT coregistered to MRI for seizure focus localization in partial epilepsy. *Mayo Clin Proc* 2000;75:615–24.
12. Yamamoto YL, Thompson CJ, Meyer E et al. Krypton-77 positron emission tomography for measurement of regional cerebral blood flow in a cross section of the head. *Acta Neurol Scand Suppl* 1977;64:448–9.
13. First International Symposium on Positron Emission Tomography. Montreal, Quebec, Canada. June 2–3, 1978. Abstracts. *J Comp Assist Tomogr* 1978;2:637–64.

14. Frackowiak RS, Lenzi GL, Jones T et al. Quantitative measurement of regional cerebral blood flow and oxygen metabolism in man using ^{15}O and positron emission tomography: theory, procedure, and normal values. *J Comp Assist Tomogr* 1980;4:727–36.

15. Connelly A, Jackson GD, Duncan JS et al. Magnetic resonance spectroscopy in temporal lobe epilepsy. *Neurology* 1994;44:1411–7.

16. Maton BM, Najm IM, Wang Y et al. Postictal *in situ* MRS brain lactate in the rat kindling model. *Neurology* 1999;53:2045–52.

17. Petroff OA, Rothman DL, Behar KL et al. Low brain GABA level is associated with poor seizure control. *Ann Neurol* 1996;40:908–11.

CHAPTER 3
Characteristic clinical and EEG findings in epilepsy syndromes

Introduction

The term "epilepsy" covers a number of different neurological syndromes resulting from epileptic activity within the brain. It is useful to classify a patient's type of epilepsy, as this may indicate the approximate location of the epileptic focus and will guide structural techniques to identify the area of abnormality. Some forms of epilepsy are related to a metabolic rather than a structural abnormality and in these cases the identification of the epileptic syndrome may help guide functional investigations. Whether the underlying abnormality is structural, metabolic, or a combination of both, identification of the syndrome type will help to determine the optimal treatment – be it surgical or medical. It will also give some idea about prognosis and allow the merits of different treatments to be compared in groups of patients with the same epilepsy syndrome.

The characteristic features that are useful for distinguishing epilepsy syndromes are discussed in this chapter. Common terms used when describing epilepsy are explained in **Table 3.1**. Syndromes that are discussed elsewhere in the book have been emphasized. To help explain the conditions described in this chapter, figures are provided indicating the positions of brain lobes and important areas within these lobes (see **Figures 3.1** and **3.2**).

Temporal lobe seizures

Temporal lobe seizures are the most common seizure type, accounting for 60%–80% of cases in surgical series. Traditionally, these seizures are divided into two groups, mesial temporal lobe seizures (MTLS) and lateral temporal lobe seizures (LTLS), on the basis that LTLS are more commonly associated with complex visual and auditory hallucinations. MTLS are more likely to be caused by hippocampal sclerosis (see **Figure 3.3**), while LTLS are more likely to be caused by tumors or areas of cortical malformation.

The majority of seizures arise within the mesial temporal lobe and begin with a visceral aura, such as a "rising" feeling in the stomach. A complex partial seizure often follows, with impaired consciousness, fixed staring, and dilated pupils. Oral automatisms may follow, such as lip-smacking, chewing, and swallowing movements. Patients may develop automatisms that either react to their surroundings semi-appropriately (reactive automatisms), or that are fixed (stereotyped automatisms). There is a postictal phase, which lasts longer if the seizure originates in the language dominant hemisphere. A typical electroencephalogram (EEG) example of a temporal lobe seizure is provided in **Figure 3.4**.

Table 3.1. Common terms used in epilepsy.

Absence attack	An episode characterized by brief staring and loss of consciousness, with few other manifestations, if any. Usually lasts less than 30 seconds
Agnosia	Inability to understand the meaning of a stimulus, usually auditory
Aphasia	Inability to form speech
Arrest reaction	Sudden rigidity or freezing of the body, sometimes in a bizarre posture
Aura	A sensation (often a strange smell or taste or a twitching in one limb), which may act as a warning that a seizure is going to happen
Automatism	Automatic or altered behavior during a complex partial seizure, which may be oral (chewing, lip-smacking), motor (rearranging objects, plucking at clothing), or other types
Axial	Affecting the trunk (as opposed to the limbs)
Hallucination	A sensation that occurs without an outside event, e.g. visual (involving vision), gustatory (involving taste)
Myoclonic jerks	Brief jerks of the whole or part of the body
Partial/generalized/ generalization	Partial seizures involve only part of the body (e.g. one limb), as opposed to generalized. Generalization describes the evolution of a seizure from a partial into a generalized one
Postictal state	Typically after a generalized seizure, a period of reduced alertness and altered behavior
Simple/complex	Simple seizures involve no loss of awareness, unlike complex seizures
Status epilepticus	When a seizure continues for a prolonged period, or when seizures occur after each other with no recovery in between
Tonic/clonic/atonic	In tonic seizures the body is held rigid, in clonic seizures there is repetitive rhythmic jerking, and in atonic seizures there is a sudden loss of muscle tone

Frontal lobe seizures

Frontal lobe seizures are the next most common seizure type, representing about 15% of cases in surgical series. Characteristic seizure types arise from several specific areas within the frontal lobe:

- supplementary motor seizures
- cingulate seizures
- anterior frontopolar seizures
- orbitofrontal seizures
- dorsolateral seizures
- opercular seizures
- motor cortex seizures

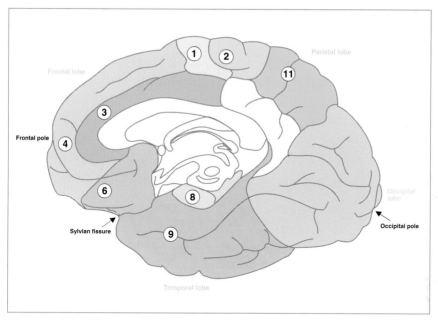

Figure 3.1. The medial surface of the right hemisphere of the brain as seen from the left (with the left hemisphere removed). 1: precentral gyrus (motor area); 2: postcentral gyrus; 3: cingulate gyrus; 4: superior frontal gyri; 6: basal frontal gyri (including orbital and olfactory gyri); 8: uncus and parahippocampal gyrus; 9: medial temporal gyri; 11: superior and inferior parietal lobules.

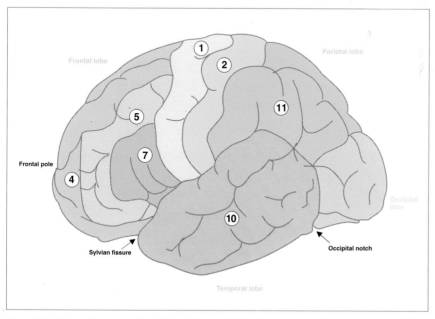

Figure 3.2. The lateral surface of the left hemisphere of the brain as seen from the left. 1: precentral gyrus (motor area); 2: postcentral gyrus; 4: superior frontal gyri; 5: middle frontal gyri; 7: inferior frontal gyri; 10: lateral temporal gyri; 11: superior and inferior parietal lobules.

R   L

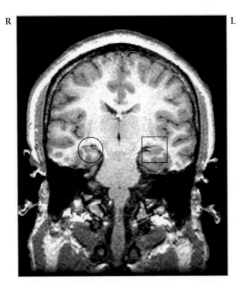

Figure 3.3. Magnetic resonance image showing right hippocampal sclerosis. The right hippocampus (circled) is smaller than the left (in the square). L: left; R: right.

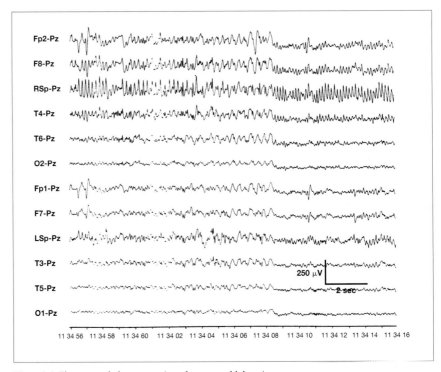

Figure 3.4. Electroencephalogram tracing of a temporal lobe seizure.

However, in practice, it is usually impossible to pinpoint the actual area where the seizure originates. Common features associated with frontal lobe seizures are:

- frequent, brief seizures that occur in clusters
- a sudden onset and offset with little or no postictal confusion
- a nocturnal predominance
- complex motor automatisms
- vocalization from simple humming to shouted expletives
- prominent mood changes
- genital or sexual automatisms
- an occasional progression to complex partial status epilepticus

Parietal lobe seizures

Parietal lobe seizures may account for up to 10% of cases in surgical series. They are relatively uncommon and are associated with multiple seizure types and patterns of spread. Unfortunately, the seizure pattern often offers no specific clinical clue as to where the seizure originates. Contralateral paresthesia (a tingling sensation on the opposite side of the body from the parietal lobe affected) was once considered typical of parietal lobe seizures but is only present in approximately 50% of patients [1]. Features suggesting a parietal lobe seizure are given in **Table 3.2.**

Table 3.2. Features suggesting parietal lobe seizures.

Parietal lobe origin	Spread to the parietal lobe
Contralateral paresthesia	Asymmetric tonic posturing
Contralateral pain	"Arrest reaction"
Gustatory hallucinations (especially parietal operculum)	Complex automatisms

Occipital lobe seizures

Occipital lobe seizures are rare. There are a wide variety of occipital seizure types, probably because there are many possible mechanisms of spread: in suprasylvian, infrasylvian, medial, and contralateral directions. However, there are some key features (usually related to the visual system) that enable recognition:

- visual hallucinations
- ictal amaurosis – a gradual fading to gray of the vision
- eye movement sensations (without detectable movement)
- tonic contralateral, or occasionally clonic, eye deviation
- prominent forced blinking or eyelid flutter

Signs of occipital lobe seizure spread are:

- focal sensory or clonic motor activity
- asymmetric tonic posturing
- visual hallucinations (which may be quite elaborate)
- automatisms like those observed in mesial temporal lobe epilepsy (occasionally)

Juvenile myoclonic epilepsy

Juvenile myoclonic epilepsy is also known as impulsive petit mal or Janz–Herpin syndrome. It first presents around the time of puberty. It is characterized in up to 88% of patients by bilateral, single, or repetitive irregular myoclonic jerks, predominantly in the arms, which are more common on awakening and after sleep deprivation. Seizures (occasionally generalized) are also associated with awakening. Some patients may fall suddenly from a jerk although there is usually no disturbance of consciousness. About 40% of these patients are photosensitive [2].

EEG findings are generalized ictal discharges of multiple spikes and slow waves. Interictally, frequent generalized bursts are observed with focal spikes, superimposed on a normal background (see **Figure 3.5**).

Childhood syndromes

Lennox–Gastaut syndrome

This syndrome usually manifests in preschool children, although it may first present in children as old as 8 years. The most common seizure types are tonic-axial, atonic, and absence attacks. Seizure frequency is generally high and status epilepticus is common. Mental retardation and delayed neurological development are also frequently observed. Children diagnosed with this condition have had a previous encephalopathy in 60% of cases.

The EEG findings are usually characterized by a slow spike-wave activity with a frequency of 1–2 Hz (see **Figure 3.6**) [3]. This is diagnostic of the condition and is often not abolished even with successful treatment of the seizures. The background EEG demonstrates generalized multiple discharges. During sleep, the EEG manifests bursts of fast rhythm activity of up to 10 Hz. Based on patterns of blood flow demonstrated using functional imaging techniques, subtypes of Lennox–Gastaut syndrome have been differentiated:

- unilateral focal
- unilateral diffuse hypometabolic
- bilateral diffuse hypometabolic
- normal

West syndrome

This condition is also known as infantile spasms or Blitz–Nick–Salaam Krampf. It usually manifests as a triad of infantile spasms, arrested psychomotor development,

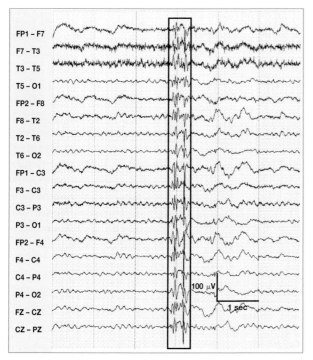

Figure 3.5. Electroencephalogram tracing showing juvenile myoclonic epilepsy. Spike discharges (in box) observed on a normal background.

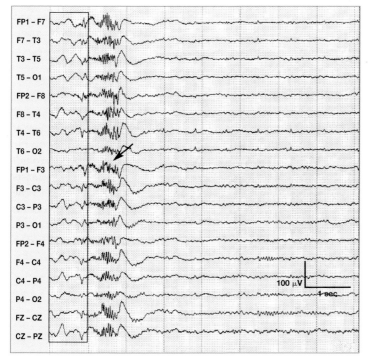

Figure 3.6. Characteristic electroencephalogram tracing showing Lennox–Gastaut syndrome. Slow spike-wave activity (in box) with generalized discharges (arrow).

and hypsarrhythmia on an EEG. Infantile spasms may be flexor, extensor, or head nods, although any combination may occur. Peak onset is between the ages of 4–7 months and the condition always presents before the age of 1 year.

Hypsarrhythmia (a high amplitude arrhythmia) manifests on the sleep EEG as a pattern of high amplitude bursts, alternating with low amplitude activity. When awake, the EEG usually has a chaotic pattern and a high voltage, with a mixture of slow activity and focal and generalized epileptiform discharges of inconstant morphology and distribution (see **Figure 3.7**). Hypsarrhythmia generally improves on the EEG with successful treatment of the seizure disorder. The onset of seizure activity is usually heralded by generalized multiple spikes and slow waves with a temporary short-lived reduction in EEG amplitude [4]. Ictal single photon emission computed tomography (SPECT) imaging has indicated that hypsarrhythmia and infantile spasms have different neurophysiological origins: hypsarrhythmia originates in the cortex and tonic spasms have a subcortical origin.

In up to a quarter of cases there is an underlying focal cerebral abnormality [5]. In these cases a good response to surgery has been reported, although, otherwise, the prognosis is generally poor.

Landau–Kleffner syndrome

Landau–Kleffner syndrome is also known as acquired epileptic aphasia. The EEG is characterized by multifocal spikes and spike-wave discharges. There is verbal auditory agnosia and a rapid reduction in spontaneous speech [6]. Seizures are usually generalized, convulsive, or partial motor in nature. Behavioral and psychomotor abnormalities occur in up to 67% of patients. Seizures tend to remit (along with EEG abnormalities) by the age of 15 years.

Sturge–Weber syndrome

Sturge–Weber syndrome (see **Figure 3.8**), also known as Sturge–Weber–Dimitri disease or encephalotrigeminal angiomatosis, is a congenital lesion that is inherited or sporadic. It is thought to be a result of abnormal vascular mesenchymal development, leading to the formation of a plexus of dilated blood vessels on the skin. This "port wine stain" is usually confined to one side of the face with a distribution following the branches of the trigeminal nerve. The skin lesion is mirrored by a plexus of immature vessels occupying the subarachnoid space of the posterior ipsilateral cerebral hemisphere, usually in the occipital or parietal regions. Blood flow changes in the underlying cerebral cortex lead to local hypoxic damage and secondary calcification, typically in a "tram-track" distribution [7]. The atrophic areas are predisposed to epileptogenic activity [8]. It has been shown that resection of the affected cortex, or even the whole hemisphere (in severe cases), is helpful for controlling epilepsy.

Tuberous sclerosis

Tuberous sclerosis (see **Figure 3.9**), also known as epiloia or Bourneville's disease, after the French physician who first described it, is a congenital disease with an autosomal dominant pattern of inheritance (although 50% of cases are caused by

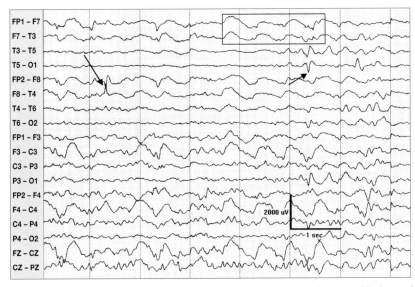

Figure 3.7. Electroencephalogram tracing showing West syndrome. Note the disorganized background with high amplitude (note scale) slowing (in box) and spikes (arrowed).

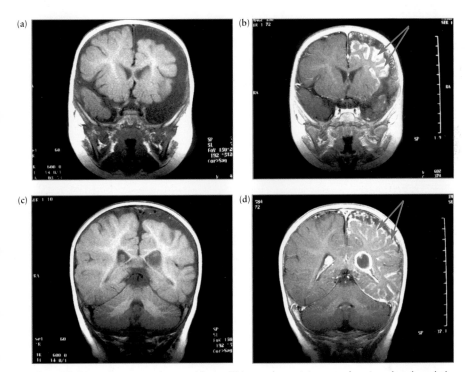

Figure 3.8. Magnetic resonance images of Sturge–Weber syndrome: (a) a coronal section taken through the anterior frontal lobe demonstrating left-sided hemiatrophy; (b) the angioma on the cortical surface enhances avidly with contrast (arrowed); (c) a similar section to (a) but taken more posteriorly in the frontal lobe, again demonstrating hemiatrophy; (d) avid enhancement of hemiatrophy with contrast (arrowed).

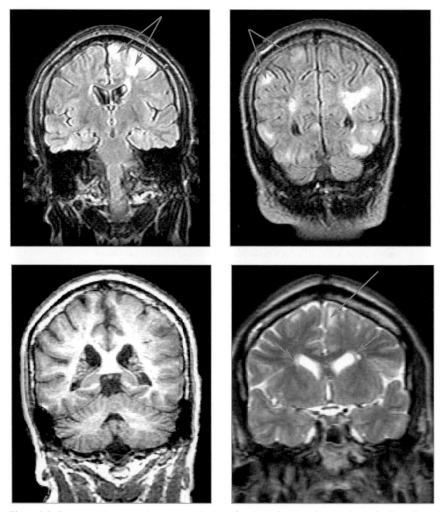

Figure 3.9. Representative magnetic resonance images showing tuberous sclerosis. Cortical tubers (long arrows) and subependymal nodules (short arrows) are demonstrated.

new mutations). Currently, diagnosis is based on the detection (using imaging criteria) of one or more brain lesions, which may take the form of a cortical hamartoma (tuber) or subependymal nodule [7,9]. These lesions are histologically identical and are thought to form as a result of a neuronal migration defect. Evidence supporting this is that cortical lesions are typically associated with disorganization of the normal laminar layers and a similar pattern of disruption is noted in the cerebellum in 20% of patients. Moreover, white matter signal abnormalities have been observed extending from the cortical tubers to the subependymal lesions.

Malformations of cortical development

Malformations of cortical development include neuronal migration disorders (NMDs) and cortical dysplasia (CD). NMDs are caused by any event that deranges the normal pattern of cortical development. During normal development, from

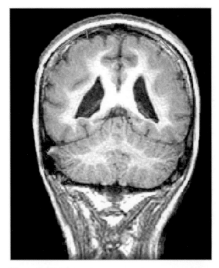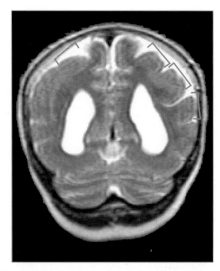

Figure 3.10. Magnetic resonance images revealing pachygyria. The abnormally thick gyri are indicated.

7 weeks' gestation onwards, cells in the subependymal layers migrate outwards (guided by radial glial fibers) towards the cerebral cortex. Subsequent waves of migration pass through the layer in which previous layers have come to rest, thereby forming an "inside-out" pattern of laminae within the cerebral cortex. With NMDs, events such as ischemia, viral infections, or genetic abnormalities act on these intricately organized processes to varying degrees, alone or in concert. Cortical malformation conditions, varying in distribution and severity, result [6,10].

Lissencephaly is a severe NMD in which the cortex is usually smooth and thickened, and the Sylvian fissures are shallow and vertically orientated. The condition is characterized by an abnormal layering of the cortex and subsequent absence of cortical folding or gyrification. Common presentations are agyria, which is an absence of gyri (the brain, or part of the brain, has a smooth surface appearance), or pachygyria, which is the presence of gyri with an abnormal thickness (see **Figure 3.10**) [11].

The etiology of lissencephaly is thought to be an NMD that occurs between 8–14 weeks' gestation. Polymicrogyria is another form of lissencephaly in which neurons successfully reach the cortex but distribute abnormally, resulting in multiple small gyri (see **Figure 3.11**).

Schizencephaly (see **Figure 3.12**) is regarded as an extreme NMD. With this condition, infolding of the cerebral cortex extends all the way to the lateral ventricle. The lips of the cleft may be fused or unfused, termed "closed lip" or "open lip", respectively.

Heterotopia is a less severe NMD in which the salient abnormality is a group (or groups) of neurons in incorrect places within the cortex. Heterotopia is usually divided morphologically into focal, diffuse, and subependymal forms. In focal heterotopia (see **Figure 3.13**) the neurons lie within the subcortical and deep white

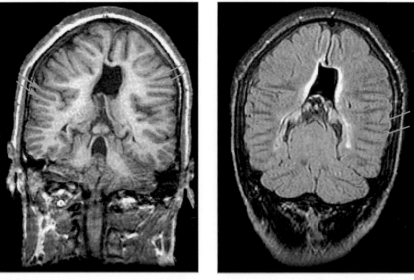

Figure 3.11. Magnetic resonance images showing polymicrogyria. Some abnormally thin gyri are indicated.

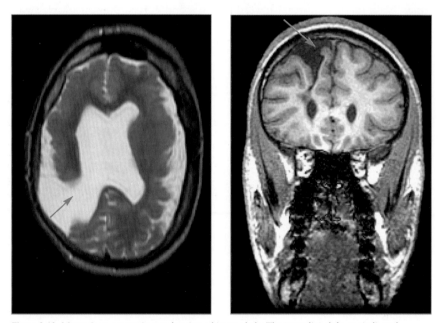

Figure 3.12. Magnetic resonance image showing schizencephaly. The (open lip) clefts are indicated.

matter. In diffuse heterotopia, the neurons may be seen as a band in a subcortical layer (sometimes leading to the appearance of "double cortex", see **Figure 3.14**). In subependymal heterotopia (see **Figure 3.15**), nodules of neurons are observed in the subependymal region that lines the lateral wall of the lateral ventricles.

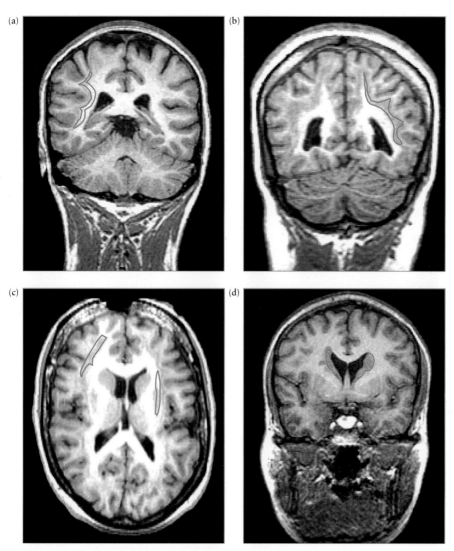

Figure 3.13. Magnetic resonance images showing focal heterotopia. The areas of heterotopia are outlined. (a–c) show band heterotopia and (d) demonstrates subependymal heterotopia.

There is debate among authors as to whether CD should be classified, along with NMDs, as a malformation of cortical development. With NMDs, migration is accomplished but the normal six-layered pattern of cortical organization is disordered, whereas CD usually presents as a focal area of abnormality in the cerebral cortex.

Megalencephaly

With megalencephaly, there is hamartomatous enlargement of either one or both sides of the brain. (The condition is termed hemimegalencephaly when only one side

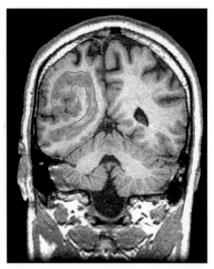

Figure 3.14. Magnetic resonance image of diffuse heterotopia showing a double cortex. The area of double cortex heterotopia is outlined.

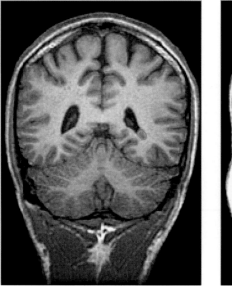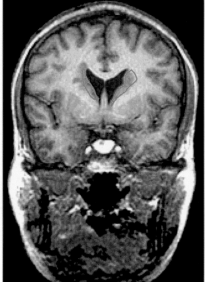

Figure 3.15. Magnetic resonance images showing subependymal heterotopia. The areas of double cortex heterotopia are outlined.

is affected.) It is usually associated with drug-resistant seizures that begin during the first few months of life. Migration abnormalities and prominent lissencephaly are usually obvious in the affected cerebral cortex.

References

1. Cascino GD, Hulihan JF, Sharbrough FW et al. Parietal lobe lesional epilepsy: electroclinical correlation and operative outcome. *Epilepsia* 1993;34:522–7.
2. Panayiotopoulos CP, Obeid T, Tahan AR. Juvenile myoclonic epilepsy: a 5 year prospective study. *Epilepsia* 1994;35:285–96.
3. Fitzgerald LF, Stone JL, Hughes JR et al. The Lennox–Gastaut syndrome: electroencephalographic characteristics, clinical correlates, and follow-up studies. *Clin Electroencephalogr* 1992;23:180–9.
4. Jacobi G, Neirich U. Symptomatology and electroencephalography of the 'genuine' type of the West syndrome and its differential diagnosis from the other benign generalized epilepsies of infancy. *Epilepsy Res Suppl* 1992;6:145–51.
5. Drury I, Beydoun A, Garofalo EA et al. Asymmetric hypsarrhythmia: clinical electroencephalographic and radiological findings. *Epilepsia* 1995;36:41–7.
6. Gordon N. The Landau–Kleffner syndrome: increased understanding. *Brain Dev* 1997;19:311–6.
7. Herron J, Darrah R, Quaghebeur G. Intracranial manifestations of the neurocutaneous syndromes. *Clin Radiol* 2000;55:82–98.
8. Westmoreland BF. The EEG findings in extratemporal seizures. *Epilepsia* 1998;39 (Suppl. 4):S1–8.
9. Sparagana SP, Roach ES. Tuberous sclerosis complex. *Curr Opin Neurol* 2000;13:115–9.
10. Andermann F. Cortical dysplasias and epilepsy: a review of the architectonic, clinical, and seizure patterns. *Adv Neurol* 2000;84:479–96.
11. Lammens M. Neuronal migration disorders in man. *Eur J Morphol* 2000;38:327–33.

CHAPTER 4
Clinical applications of functional imaging

Introduction
In this chapter the current uses of functional imaging are discussed, paying particular attention to:

- localization of occult foci
- preoperative localization of functionally important tissue (especially speech and motor centers)
- imaging levels of brain neurotransmitters, such as gamma-aminobutyric acid (GABA)
- functional imaging in the assessment of neurotoxicity
- imaging of specific epilepsy syndromes

These topics of research are specifically related to epilepsy treatment and diagnosis, and are areas where functional imaging can provide useful information over and above that obtainable using the currently available structural and electrographic techniques.

Localization of occult foci
Several functional techniques have been shown to be useful in cases where structural imaging or electroencephalography (EEG) fail to reveal an identifiable abnormality.

Functional MRI
As discussed in Chapter 2, recent technological advances have made EEG triggering of functional magnetic resonance imaging (fMRI) possible. It has been shown that this technique can be performed safely in a scanning environment. Triggering of the fMRI scan by interictal discharges allows visualization of the cortical area that is involved in the initiation of seizures – the irritative zone. Since studies have shown that the distribution of interictal spikes is a good predictor of the outcome after surgical resection [1], the irritative zone is thought to be closely related to the epileptogenic zone. There may even be advantages in identifying the irritative zone rather than the area of seizure spread. An example of an EEG-triggered BOLD (blood oxygenation level dependent) scan identifying an epileptic focus is provided in **Figure 4.1**. Another example showing a BOLD activation superimposed onto a 3-dimensional representation of a brain is provided in **Figure 4.2**.

EEG-triggered fMRI provides useful information in patients with epilepsy arising from various localized pathologies, including hippocampal sclerosis, dysembryoplastic neuroepithelial tumor, astrocytoma, cortical dysgenesis, and chronic encephalitis [2]. As this technology improves, it will soon become possible to obtain useful localizing information in patients in whom no structural imaging abnormality is found.

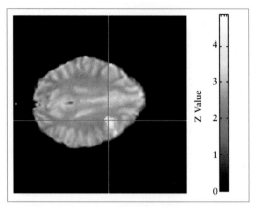

Figure 4.1. Example of an electroencephalography-triggered blood oxygenation level dependent (BOLD) activation. The Z value relates to the probability of an area being active (as in a statistical parametric map [SPM]). An active focus is demonstrated in the left frontal lobe. The image is courtesy of Dr M Symms, National Society of Epilepsy.

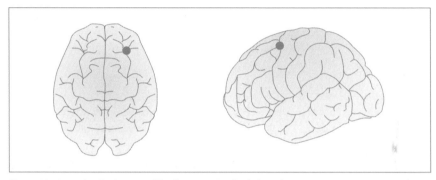

Figure 4.2. Area of activation on a blood oxygenation level dependent (BOLD) scan superimposed onto a 3-dimensional representation of a brain.

SPECT

Single photon emission computed tomography (SPECT) is a highly sensitive technique for detecting occult foci. Ictal injection of technetium-99m-D,L-hexamethylpropyleneamineoxime ($^{99}Tc^m$-HMPAO) is more valuable than interictal or postictal injection. In 70% or more of cases of temporal and extratemporal epilepsy, the focus has been accurately identified using SPECT [3]. Surgical series have demonstrated the value of SPECT for identifying resectable lesions.

SPECT has also been used in cingulate gyrus epilepsy. San Pedro et al. documented the case of a patient in whom a focus could not be identified using a surface EEG because of the relatively deep location of the gyrus and the rapid occurrence of widespread seizure propagation almost immediately after seizure onset [4]. Using SPECT, a focus in the anterior cingulate gyrus was identified and the seizure pattern was subsequently characterized using subdural electrodes. Surgical resection resulted in a greater than 90% reduction in seizure frequency. A SPECT image identifying a previously unsuspected focus in the anterior portion of the right frontal lobe cortex is provided in **Figure 4.3**. **Figure 4.4** demonstrates right hippocampal sclerosis (observed on an MR image) with right temporal lobe interictal hypoperfusion and ictal hyperperfusion.

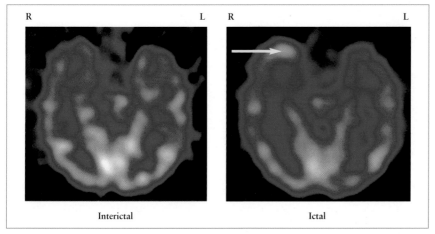

Figure 4.3. An unsuspected ictal focus shown on a SPECT scan (arrow): (a) interictal SPECT scan showing symmetrical activity; (b) ictal SPECT scan. L: left; R: right; SPECT: single photon emission computed tomography. This figure is courtesy of Professor I Gordon.

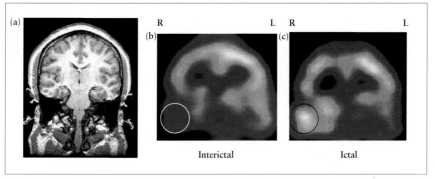

Figure 4.4. SPECT image showing hippocampal sclerosis: (a) MR scan; (b) interictal SPECT scan showing right temporal lobe hypoperfusion (circled); (c) ictal SPECT scan showing right temporal lobe hyperperfusion (circled). L: left; MR: magnetic resonance; R: right; SPECT: single photon emission computed tomography. This figure is courtesy of Professor I Gordon.

PET

Using ^{18}F-fluoro-deoxyglucose (^{18}F-FDG) positron emission tomography (PET), hypometabolism has been detected in the affected area in 90% of cases of temporal lobe epilepsy due to mesial temporal (hippocampal) sclerosis [5]. In cases of extratemporal or lateral temporal (neocortical) epilepsy, the rate of regional hypometabolism is lower, approximately 70%. PET has also demonstrated a highly focal decrease in central benzodiazepine receptor (cBZR) density in hippocampal sclerosis [6], although the structural abnormality is usually evident using high-quality MRI. In some cases, ^{11}C-flumazenil PET is more specific (although less sensitive) than ^{18}F-FDG PET, since the former images neuronal density and the latter may reflect reduced glucose activity due to diaschisis. Diaschisis is the term used to describe reduced metabolic activity in a neural pathway that is connected to an area that has been damaged, e.g. by a stroke. **Figure 4.5** illustrates the histological (using autoradiography of flumazenil receptors) confirmation of *in vivo* PET scans

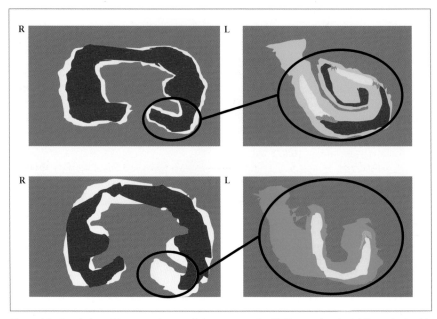

Figure 4.5. Correlation of *in vivo* positron emission tomography (PET) scans (on the left) in patients with and without hippocampal sclerosis with autoradiography of resected specimens (on the right). The upper images (patients without hippocampal sclerosis) demonstrate normal PET scans with symmetrical uptake of tracer (shown in red) in both temporal lobes and normal autoradiography of the magnified left temporal lobe with normal cell layers colored according to concentration from yellow to red. The lower images (patients with hippocampal sclerosis) demonstrate a decrease in activity in the left temporal lobe on PET (circled) with loss of normal hippocampal cell layers on autoradiography. These data are courtesy of Dr A Hammers, National Society of Epilepsy. L: left; R: right.

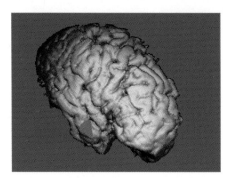

Figure 4.6. Positron emission tomography (PET) scan showing the area of increased uptake in the right temporal lobe cortex superimposed onto a 3-dimensional brain reconstruction.

in patients with and without hippocampal sclerosis. **Figure 4.6** illustrates the positive identification of an area of increased ictal activity in the right temporal lobe cortex using ^{18}F-FDG PET. An MR scan was normal in this patient.

MRS

Magnetic resonance spectroscopy (MRS) has been used to monitor metabolic changes in the affected lobe in temporal lobe epilepsy, involving variations in the levels of *N*-acetyl aspartate (NAA), choline (Cho), and creatine (Cr) resulting in a decrease in the NAA/(Cho+Cr) ratio. This is thought to reflect loss of or damage to neurons with a corresponding increase in gliosis. These changes have been demonstrated in both adults and children and have been shown to accord with extensive EEG investigation in up to 99% of patients with temporal lobe epilepsy [7]. Recently, using the NAA/(Cho+Cr) ratio, ^{1}H MRS has been used to detect metabolic abnormalities in patients with temporal lobe epilepsy who have normal MR scans [8].

In neocortical temporal lobe epilepsy, where the epileptogenic lesion is thought to reside in the temporal neocortex and not the hippocampal region, multislice ^{1}H chemical shift imaging (CSI) has demonstrated that the hippocampi are indeed normal and that the metabolic abnormality resides in the cortex of the symptomatic temporal lobe and occasionally the adjacent frontal lobe [9].

With the availability of CSI, which allows larger volumes to be sampled, it has become possible to detect areas of metabolic abnormality in extratemporal regions [10]. The most marked area of metabolic abnormality was found to be in the region of the seizure focus. Other studies have demonstrated metabolic changes in unaffected parts of the frontal lobe in patients with frontal lobe epilepsy [11,12]. [31]P spectroscopy can be used to locate frontal lobe foci.

MRS can be used to detect neuronal dysfunction. Li et al. found that nearly 50% of patients with localized epilepsy had areas of abnormality corresponding to neuronal dysfunction that were larger than the areas identified by structural imaging techniques or electrographic assessment [13].

GABA imaging
Brain GABA levels correlate with seizure control. Moreover, using MRS, changes in the GABA level caused by anticonvulsants can be monitored noninvasively. As this field develops, the ability to titrate a patient's dose according to chemical criteria, rather than on the basis of symptom relief, will become possible. However, much work needs to be done before the exact role of GABA in the brain can be determined.

Diffusion-weighted MRI
This is a promising technique for identifying occult areas of abnormality in several different parts of the brain in patients with epilepsy. Studies have shown that areas of cortical dysgenesis have abnormal values on diffusion-weighted images. In addition, changes in diffusivity have been located in the frontal lobe of patients with nocturnal frontal lobe epilepsy [14]. It is likely that these changes represent areas of cortical dysplasia with an associated alteration in the macromolecular structure. As this technique, and the parallel technique of magnetization transfer imaging, advance, it should become possible to image dysgenetic lesions that are occult on conventional structural MR scans.

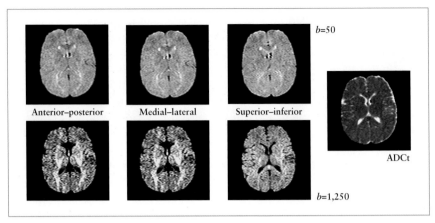

Figure 4.7. Matched images are shown, with mainly T2-weighted images (b=50) being compared with heavily diffusion-weighted images (b=1,250). It can be seen that the anterior–posterior and medial–lateral axes emphasize the tracts of the internal capsule, while the superior–inferior axis emphasizes the fibers in the forceps minor. ADCt is a composite image derived from diffusion measurements in different axes. ADC: apparent diffusion coefficient. This figure is courtesy of Philips Medical.

Diffusion imaging changes, probably reflecting changes in the cellular structure, have been demonstrated in hippocampi that appear sclerotic using MR criteria. With future refinements this technique will become more sensitive and should provide extra supporting evidence for the presence of hippocampal sclerosis where structural correlation is equivocal or even absent.

Since diffusion preferentially occurs along the length of axons in normal neural tissue, diffusion-weighted magnetic resonance imaging (dwMRI) has been used to map the normal neural tracts in the gray and white matter (tractography). An example of a dwMRI study of a neurologically normal volunteer in whom the three orthogonal axes – posterior–anterior, medial–lateral, and superior–inferior – are studied with diffusivity in each direction being calculated is provided in **Figure 4.7**. The tracts running in each axis are emphasized. Neurosurgical procedures can be planned using dwMRI because tumors and dysgenetic lesions distort the surrounding functional pathways and there is considerable variation in the course of tracts. Important motor pathways may be mapped and avoided, thus reducing the risk that epilepsy surgery will cause a neurological deficit.

Preoperative localization of functionally important tissue

This promising application of functional imaging has been used to map important areas, such as the motor strip or those areas involved in language, prior to epilepsy surgery. Some examples of activations in healthy volunteers are illustrated in **Figure 4.8**. The importance of preoperative mapping of eloquent regions of cortex is particularly pressing in epilepsy patients, for a number of reasons:

- Studies have demonstrated an increased variability of hemispheric language representation in patients with epilepsy.

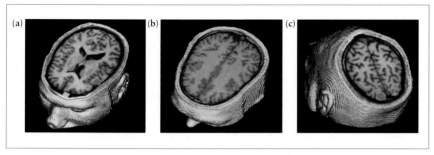

Figure 4.8. Examples of activations measured using functional magnetic resonance imaging: (a) verbal fluency; (b) recall task; and (c) checkerboard. This figure is courtesy of Philips Medical.

- Patients undergoing cortical resection for epilepsy may have structural cortical disorders, such as dysplasia or tumors, which have a mass effect. The usual representation of neurological function on the cortical surface may be altered.
- Patients with epilepsy may have suffered a vascular or metabolic event early in life, leading to infarction of a cortical area. Unexpected areas of the cortex may have taken over important neurological functions.

Traditionally, if there is concern that an epileptogenic lesion is within or very close to an eloquent area, intracranial stimulation (ICS) studies are performed using subdurally implanted electrodes. These electrodes can be electrically stimulated to determine the function supplied by the underlying cortex. ICS studies are usually performed at surgery and require direct visualization of the cortex through a craniotomy to see where, anatomically, the electrode is being placed.

Functional studies have several advantages over ICS studies[15]:

- The patient has a smaller craniotomy (only the region to be resected). The whole cortex can be studied using functional techniques, whereas the area that can be examined using ICS studies is limited by the size of the craniotomy.
- There is a reduced operating time. Using functional techniques the surgeon has a clear idea of the cortical region that needs to be resected. ICS studies can be extremely time consuming in difficult cases.
- The procedure is more tolerable to the patient. ICS studies require that the patient is awakened after the craniotomy to cooperate with testing of cortical activities; understandably, some patients find this distressing.
- Since functional studies are coregistered with high-resolution MR scans, they may allow easier identification of the cortical abnormality requiring resection, especially when the cortical anatomy itself is abnormal due to dysplasia or distortion from tumor or mass effect.
- In some cases, ICS studies may precipitate seizures, which can make identification of the spontaneously epileptogenic region difficult.
- They can be repeated more easily in cases where the initial results are unclear or considered atypical because they allow assessment to be performed with no surgical risk.

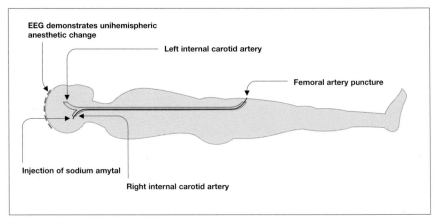

EEG demonstrates unihemispheric anesthetic change

Left internal carotid artery

Femoral artery puncture

Injection of sodium amytal

Right internal carotid artery

Figure 4.9. Illustration of the Wada test: each internal carotid artery is catheterized in turn and injected with sodium amytal, which temporarily anesthetizes the hemisphere. During this time the other hemisphere is tested for language and memory functions. EEG: electroencephalogram.

However, functional tests have some disadvantages when compared to ICS studies:

- Most require cooperation with an experimental paradigm, necessitating the patient's comprehension and attentiveness (which may particularly be a limiting factor in children).
- Images are considerably degraded by movement, particularly with fMRI. The patient must stay still, which can be difficult using some paradigms and for children.

Language lateralization in the temporal lobe prior to lobectomy
Temporal lobe epilepsy due to hippocampal sclerosis is a common pathology for which there is a successful surgical treatment – temporal lobectomy. However, removal of the language dominant temporal lobe (i.e. the side of the brain that produces and understands language) is associated with risks to language function and verbal memory.

A Wada test is usually performed to determine the dominant hemisphere (see **Figure 4.9**). This involves the patient having a cerebral angiogram, during which a femoral artery puncture is made, a catheter is passed up into each internal carotid artery in turn, and injections of sodium amytal (a short-acting barbiturate) are made, anesthetizing each hemisphere. During the few minutes that the amytal has anesthetized one hemisphere, the other hemisphere is tested for language and memory function.

Although widely used, the Wada test does have some associated difficulties:

- In some cases it is difficult to avoid the phenomenon of "crossflow", whereby amytal passes over to the contralateral hemisphere via the circle of Willis. This hinders the neurological assessment of the ipsilateral hemisphere.

- The anesthetization of the hemisphere in question may not be complete during the entire testing period (the amytal is administered as a bolus injection, which gradually wears off).
- Testing is limited to a short time frame, typically a few minutes per hemisphere, and cannot be repeated (or extended) without the patient undergoing the invasive procedure again.
- Because of potential morbidity associated with the Wada test, results from healthy control subjects are lacking. Our understanding and interpretation of the test are therefore mainly based on patients suffering from neurological disorders.
- Catheterization of the internal carotid artery carries a small but important risk of stroke, and femoral artery puncture is associated with a risk of hematoma, which may be painful.

Functional imaging paradigms have been developed to replace and extend the language function examination carried out by the Wada test. There is still some debate regarding the most specific paradigm for identification of cortical areas responsible for language, since fMRI is extremely sensitive and will also pick up areas that are activated by association and are not directly responsible for language processing. However, a paradigm described by Binder et al. demonstrated a 96% correlation with the Wada test ($P<0.0001$) [16]. The test involved was a single word semantic decision task.

Subjects were scanned with their eyes closed in a darkened room. Stimuli used were digitally synthesized aural tones or sampled male speech sounds, presented binaurally. The stimuli were sent to the subjects via air conduction through plastic tubes, which were threaded through tightly occlusive ear inserts. Therefore, the background scanner noise was kept at a constant level.

The paradigm consisted of a pair of tasks whose cerebral activations were compared. The first task was designed to stimulate the subject's attention to the physical characteristics of an auditory stimulus – "tone decision". A short sequence of pure synthesizer tones of either 500 or 750 Hz was presented and the subject was asked to respond if any of the sequences contained two or more 750 Hz tones. The second task was designed to direct attention to semantic information related to linguistic stimuli – "semantic decision". For this task, the stimuli were spoken English nouns representing animals. No animal name was used twice. Subjects were asked to respond if they considered the animal to be both "native to the US" and "used by humans". Responses were made by thumb pressing a button device held in the left hand. Both stimuli were presented to the subject a number of times. The subjects were given practice runs before scanning actually started.

Activation from the first task was subtracted from activation from the second task to yield the activation due to language alone. In the first task, it was hypothesized that a variety of nonlinguistic functional systems would be activated, including attention arousal, sensory processing, short-term processing, and motor systems. In the second task, the nonlinguistic functional systems as well as the linguistic systems would be activated. Therefore, the rationale was that subtraction of the two tasks would yield imaging of linguistic functional systems alone.

Postprocessing was performed to control for the effects of head movement. Activation data were geometrically transformed into a standardized space to facilitate intersubject comparison.

Using this paradigm, it was found that the language area, as might be expected, localized mainly to areas around the superior temporal sulcus in the dominant hemisphere. Activation also spread ventrally across parts of the inferior temporal gyrus and the fusiform and parahippocampal gyri in the ventral temporal lobe. However, three other distinct areas were also activated:

- a prefrontal region, including the inferior and superior frontal gyri, and rostral and caudal aspects of the middle frontal gyrus
- the dominant angular gyrus
- a perisplenic region including the posterior cingulate, ventromedial precuneus, and cingulate isthmus

The prefrontal region is thought to play an executive language role, co-coordinating sensory and semantic processes and incorporating instant changes in goals and strategy. The perisplenic region is thought to be connected to hippocampal and parahippocampal regions and may therefore play a role in memory functions.

Motor and sensory mapping prior to neurosurgery

Encouraging results have indicated that fMRI can reliably locate the motor strip to an accuracy of within 1.7 mm (this has been verified by intraoperative electrographic studies). With additional information from PET imaging studies, this disparity can be reduced to 1.2 mm [17,18]. The visual cortex has also been mapped functionally, again with a high degree of accuracy [19].

Motor functions generally induce larger blood flow changes than cognitive functions. The movement of a finger or toe results in a blood flow change of 5%–6% whereas a 1%–2% change is detected with a cognitive function. This gives paradigms for motor mapping an advantage over cognitive paradigms. Sensory paradigms produce an intermediate change and are varied, but generally include tactile stimulation of a body part, e.g. the tongue (see **Figure 4.10**).

Imaging of brain GABA levels

At present, studies of brain GABA levels have yielded conflicting results. GABA is involved in elaborate and interconnected processes; therefore, measurements are only wide-ranging estimates. The future aim is to obtain meaningful measurements that can be interpreted. Results from preliminary research are promising: a recent study of children with epilepsy has demonstrated an increase in brain GABA levels (as measured by MRS) in the age group between 1 and 5 years old [20].

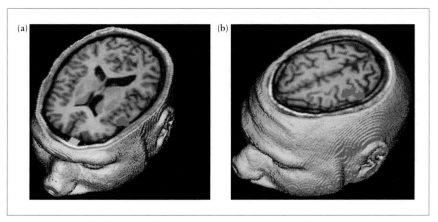

Figure 4.10. Examples of motor and sensory activations using functional magnetic resonance imaging: (a) lateral tongue; (b) finger tapping. This figure is courtesy of Philips Medical.

Topiramate, vigabatrin, and gabapentin (antiepileptic drugs) all increase brain GABA levels in patients with epilepsy [21,22]. In the future, direct imaging of brain GABA levels in these patients will guide the choice of drug and determine the dosage that should be used for treatment.

Functional imaging in the assessment of neurotoxicity

To help elucidate the mechanisms of drug action and toxicity, PET has been used to gauge the effect of various anticonvulsants on regional cerebral glucose metabolism (see **Table 4.1**).

Table 4.1. The effect of various anticonvulsants on regional cerebral glucose metabolism.

Anticonvulsant	Mean overall reduction in cerebral glucose metabolism	Regions most affected
Barbiturates	37%	Global
Phenytoin	13%	Frontal and parietal
Carbamazepine	12%	Superior frontal
Valproate	22%	Global

Further studies are necessary, but soon it may be possible to use functional imaging to gain an insight into the mechanisms of anticonvulsant neurotoxicity, which may lead to the development of new drugs with improved safety profiles.

Imaging of specific syndromes
Absence seizures
It has been known for a long time that the administration of opioids is associated with an increase in the general spike-wave EEG activity, whereas endogenous

opioids are associated with anticonvulsant effects. These findings implicate opioids in the pathogenesis of absence seizures. Recently, it has been found that genetic variation in the mu opioid receptor is linked to idiopathic absence epilepsy [23]. Therefore, future research will concentrate on imaging of opioid receptor agonists and antagonists (probably with PET and SPECT imaging) in an attempt to determine how they vary in patients with absence seizures. At present PET scanning is usually normal in absence epilepsy, although a generalized hypermetabolism may be evident if seizures are frequent. However, in the future, this technique may become a clinically valuable tool for diagnosing and assessing these patients.

Malformations of cortical development

Studies have shown that malformations of cortical development (MCD) have abnormal values on a diffusion-weighted MR scan. Dysgenetic tissue has a lower density than the surrounding gray matter (as indicated by a higher mean diffusion coefficient) and a lower degree of structural organization than the surrounding white matter (as indicated by a lower anisotropy) [24]. Interestingly, these differences are not visible on standard MR images. This finding has prompted the development of more sophisticated sequences that will define areas of MCD more sensitively and specifically.

MCD have many different appearances and can be difficult to visualize using MRI. After treatment, patients with epilepsy and MCD do not fare as well as patients with other types of lesions (only 20%–40% of these patients become seizure free, compared to 70% of patients with hippocampal sclerosis). It is thought that one reason for this is that the anatomical and functional abnormality may be more extensive than observed on the MR scan. Therefore, the abnormal area may be incompletely resected if only MRI is used for diagnosis. Using functional imaging techniques the extent of the lesion can be completely identified.

Supporting evidence for this theory comes from studies using statistical parametric map (SPM) analysis of cBZR concentration with ^{11}C-flumazenil PET, coregistered with MR. These studies have shown that more extensive abnormal areas are frequently visualized than previously appreciated, and in some cases abnormal tissue may be detected a distance from the site of the abnormality that is visualized by MR [25]. An example in which a minor malformation of cortical development was correlated with a focus using ^{11}C-flumazenil PET is provided in **Figure 4.11**. Further work has shown that flumazenil binding is increased in cortex overlying areas of band heterotopia and polymicrogyria (see **Figures 4.12** and **4.13**).

Lissencephaly and hemimegalencephaly

Some interesting findings have already been reported in patients with lissencephaly and hemimegalencephaly. Using SPECT, Chiron et al. have shown that children with lissencephaly type I (also known as agyria-pachygyria) combined with infantile spasms show differences in regional cerebral blood flow when compared to age-matched controls (especially in the age group under 3 years old) [26]. This difference in blood flow was not found in infantile spasm patients without a demonstrable cortical malformation. These findings imply that SPECT can detect changes in blood flow that are associated with evolving cortical malformations.

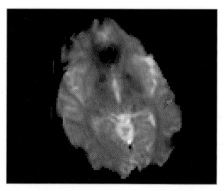

Figure 4.11. Positron emission tomography image demonstrating increased flumazenil binding in a small malformation of cortical development. The area of increased uptake is shown in red. This figure is courtesy of Dr M Symms, National Society of Epilepsy.

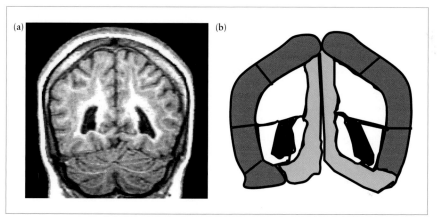

Figure 4.12. Demonstration of increased flumazenil binding in band heterotopia: (a) magnetic resonance (MR) scan; (b) ^{11}C-flumazenil positron emission tomography with an area of abnormal uptake shown in red. This area overlays the band heterotopia. These data are courtesy of Dr A Hammers, National Society of Epilepsy.

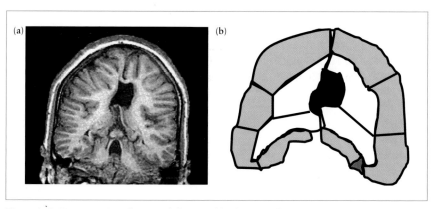

Figure 4.13. Demonstration of increased flumazenil binding in polymicrogyria: (a) magnetic resonance scan; (b) ^{11}C-flumazenil positron emission tomography image with an area of abnormal uptake shown in red. This area is adjacent to the area of polymicrogyria. These data are courtesy of Dr A Hammers, National Society of Epilepsy.

Using MRS to investigate hemimegalencephaly, a disorder characterized by an enlarged hemisphere with an associated moderate or severe malformation of cortical development, has revealed interesting results. In the affected hemisphere, there is a dramatic reduction in the levels of NAA and glutamate in the white matter, which reflects a loss of neuroaxonal tissue. This is not observed in the cortex, basal ganglia, or cerebellum. In the gray matter, increases in the levels of inositol and Cho have been observed, which reflects gliosis [27].

Lennox–Gastaut syndrome

PET scanning demonstrates regional or multiregional hypometabolism in up to 90% of patients with this condition. Functional imaging has helped to differentiate various subtypes of Lennox–Gastaut syndrome on the basis of patterns of altered blood flow. Not enough is yet known about how each subtype responds to medical and/or surgical treatment but as this information becomes available, we should be in a better position to determine the optimal therapy for each subgroup.

West syndrome

PET has identified metabolic abnormalities in many cases of previously "cryptogenic" infantile spasms. Studies of children with infantile spasms have found high degrees of abnormalities of glucose metabolism; the majority of these correspond to focal ictal or interictal EEG abnormalities. Furthermore, if a single region of abnormal glucose metabolism is identified using PET (approximately 20% of cases), and the seizures are intractable, surgical removal of the PET focus not only results in seizure control but also in complete or partial reversal of the associated developmental delay.

Functional imaging has indicated that different parts of the brain are responsible for the different characteristic symptoms of West syndrome – hypsarrhythmia is thought to arise from the cortex whereas infantile spasms appear to be generated from a subcortical focus. In addition, blood flow studies using PET have indicated that increased flow is probably reflected in a continued generalized seizure activity, whereas decreased flow is associated with the underlying cortical lesion [28].

Tuberous sclerosis

PET has been used to identify epileptogenic tubers in tuberous sclerosis (TS). With TS, a large number of tubers may be visible using structural imaging techniques. Resection of some of these tubers is associated with a reduction in seizure frequency but it is difficult to identify the tubers that should be resected. Using glucose PET, nonspecific accumulation has been observed in both epileptogenic and nonepileptogenic tubers. However, Juhasz et al. have described the use of α-^{11}C-methyl-L-tryptophan (^{11}C-AMT) to specifically detect epileptic foci [29]. This tracer was designed to measure the rate of *in vivo* synthesis of 5-hydroxytryptamine (5-HT), because intravenously injected ^{11}C-AMT is converted into ^{11}C-5-HT in the brain. ^{11}C-5-HT accumulates in nerve terminals, since it is not metabolized.

Sturge–Weber syndrome

Most cases of Sturge–Weber syndrome (SWS) are associated with partial seizures, although some patients have generalized seizures or no seizures at all. PET has revealed a unilateral diffuse hypometabolism, ipsilateral to the facial nevus, which extends beyond the abnormality that has been detected using structural imaging techniques. Furthermore, a pattern of increased glucose utilization has been demonstrated in the cerebral cortex of the anatomically affected hemisphere in children with SWS and a recent onset of epilepsy [28]. Metabolism correlates with progressive neuronal dysfunction.

In some patients with SWS and epilepsy that is difficult to control, PET has been used to guide cortical resection and assess the suitability of the patient for early hemispherectomy.

References

1. Ebersole JS, Wade PB. Spike voltage topography identifies two types of frontotemporal epileptic foci. *Neurology* 1991;41:1425–33.
2. Krakow K, Woermann FG, Symms R et al. EEG triggered functional MRI of interictal epileptiform activity in patients with partial seizures. *Brain* 1999;122:1679–88.
3. Newton MR, Berkovic SF, Austin MC et al. SPECT in the localisation of extratemporal and temporal seizure foci. *J Neurol Neurosurg Psychiatry* 1995;59:26–30
4. San Pedro EC, Mountz JM, Ojha B et al. Anterior cingulate gyrus epilepsy: the role of ictal rCBF SPECT in seizure localization. *Epilepsia* 2000;41:594–600.
5. Spencer SS, Theodore WH, Berkovic SF. Clinical applications: MRI, SPECT, and PET. *Magn Reson Imaging* 1995;13:1119-24.
6. Koepp MJ, Richardson MP, Brooks DJ et al. Cerebral benzodiazepine receptors in hippocampal sclerosis. An objective *in vivo* analysis. *Brain* 1996;119:1677–87.
7. Cendes F, Caramanos Z, Andermann F et al. Proton magnetic resonance spectroscopic imaging and magnetic resonance imaging volumetry in the lateralisation of temporal lobe epilepsy: a series of 100 patients. *Ann Neurol* 2000;42:737–46.
8. Connelly A, van Paesschen W, Porter DA et al. Proton magnetic resonance spectroscopy in MRI-negative temporal lobe epilepsy. *Neurology* 1998;51:61–6.
9. Vermathen P, Ende G, Laxer KD et al. Hippocampal N-acetyl aspartate in neocortical epilepsy and mesial temporal lobe epilepsy. *Ann Neurol* 1997;42:194–9.
10. Stanley JA, Cendes F, Dubeau F et al. Proton magnetic resonance spectroscopic imaging in patients with extratemporal epilepsy. *Epilepsia* 1998;39:267–73.
11. Garcia PA, Laxer KD, Ng T. Application of spectroscopic imaging in epilepsy. *Mag Reson Imaging* 1995;13:1181–5.
12. Garcia PA, Laxer KD, van der Grond J et al. Phosphorus magnetic resonance spectroscopic imaging in patients with frontal lobe epilepsy. *Ann Neurol* 1994;35:217–21.
13. Li LM, Cendes F, Andermann F et al. Spatial extent of neuronal metabolic dysfunction measured by proton MR spectroscopic imaging in patients with localization-related epilepsy. *Epilepsia* 2000;41:666–74.
14. Ferini Strambi L, Bozzali M, Cercignani M et al. Magnetization transfer and diffusion-weighted imaging in nocturnal frontal lobe epilepsy. *Neurology* 2000;54:2331–3.
15. Bittar RG, Olivier A, Sadikot AF et al. Presurgical motor and somatosensory cortex mapping with functional magnetic resonance imaging and positron emission tomography. *J Neurosurg* 1999;91:915–21.
16. Binder JR, Swanson SJ, Hammeke TA et al. Determination of language dominance using functional MRI: a comparison with the Wada test. *Neurology* 1996;46:978–84.

17. Braun V, Dempf S, Tomczak R et al. Multimodal cranial neuronavigation: direct integration of functional magnetic resonance imaging and positron emission tomography data: technical note. *Neurosurg* 2001;48:1178–81 [discussion 1181–2].

18. Baumann SB, Noll DC, Kondziolka DS et al. Comparison of functional magnetic resonance imaging with positron emission tomography and magnetoencephalography to identify the motor cortex in a patient with an arteriovenous malformation. *J Image Guid Surg* 1995;1:191–7.

19. Mora BN, Carman GJ, Allman JM. *In vivo* functional localization of the human visual cortex using positron emission tomography and magnetic resonance imaging. *Trends Neurosci* 1989;12:282–4.

20. Novotny EJ Jr, Hyder F, Shevell MI et al. GABA changes with vigabatrin in the developing human brain. *Epilepsia* 1999;40:462–6.

21. Petroff OAC, Rothman DL, Behar KL et al. Initial observations of the effect of gabapentin on brain GBA in patients with epilepsy. *Ann Neurol* 1996;39:95–9.

22. Petroff OAC, Rothman DL, Behar KL et al. Localized ¹H NMR measurements of gamma aminobutyric acid in human brain *in vivo*. *Proc Natl Acad Sci USA* 1993;15:5662–6.

23. Sander T, Berlin W, Gscheidel N et al. Genetic variation of the human mu opioid receptor and susceptibility to idiopathic absence epilepsy. *Epilepsy Res* 2000;39:57–61.

24. Krakow K, Wieshmann U, Woermann FG et al. Multimodal MR imaging: functional, diffusion tensor, and chemical shift imaging in a patient with localisation related epilepsy. *Epilepsia* 1999;40:1459–62.

25. Richardson MP, Koepp MJ, Brooks DJ et al. Cerebral activation in malformations of cortical development. *Brain* 1998;121:1295–304.

26. Chiron C, Nabbout R, Pinton F et al. Brain functional imaging SPECT in agyria-pachygyria. *Epilepsy Res* 1996;24:109–17.

27. Hanefeld F, Kruse B, Holzbach U et al. Hemimegalencephaly: localized proton magnetic resonance spectroscopy *in vivo*. *Epilepsia* 1995;36:1215–24.

28. Chugani HT, Chugani DC. Basic mechanisms of childhood epilepsies: studies with positron emission tomography. *Adv Neurol* 1999;79:883–91.

29. Juhasz C, Chugani DC, Muzik O et al. Relationship between EEG and positron emission tomography abnormalities in clinical epilepsy. *J Clin Neurophysiol* 2000;17:29–42.

CHAPTER 5
Future developments

The future of epilepsy research and treatment is exciting. Technical advances will allow important information to be gained regarding the pathophysiology of epilepsy. Consequently, our ability to confidently diagnose the source of a patient's epilepsy will improve, particularly when the combined data from functional studies, high-resolution structural imaging, and neurophysiological studies, such as electroencephalography, are considered.

Medical and surgical advances will enhance our ability to treat epilepsy. The receptor status (i.e. the number of receptors for important neurochemicals, such as gamma-aminobutyric acid, and the proportion that are occupied at one time) of a patient for various neurotransmitters involved in epilepsy will become more easily assessable and interpretable. This will result in targeted drug treatments and a better titration of anticonvulsants, which will reduce side effects and toxicity. With a better knowledge of drug action, new drugs will be developed to target receptors more specifically. New receptors may be identified, which may then be manipulated to improve medical therapy, and monitoring of drug treatment (in terms of receptor density and binding) will soon be possible. A clearer understanding of the functional anatomy underlying each patient's seizure disorder will result in a more targeted neurosurgical intervention in selected cases.

Using functional magnetic resonance imaging (fMRI), the following improvements may be envisaged as our experience increases:

- The paradigms used to define areas involved in specific functions – such as motor tasks or speech – will improve.
- New MR sequences will be developed, generating better contrast and spatial resolutions.
- Improvements in hardware – with better head coils and more homogeneous magnetic fields – will also help to enhance contrast and spatial resolutions.

With magnetic resonance spectroscopy, increased strength and homogeneity of the magnetic field, as well as improvements in signal postprocessing, will facilitate signal characterization from different molecular species. Also, with diffusion-weighted imaging, which is currently in its infancy, the development of more sophisticated software will enable delineation of complicated neural pathways: visualization of neural tracts – "tractography" – is already becoming possible.

With the impending improvements in MR-based functional images, an eventual convergence of techniques can be predicted, with an fMRI examination being carried out in a single, extended session. As a result of software and hardware improvements and advances in knowledge about the sensitivity, specificity, and reproducibility of the various techniques available, the functional examination could be carried out more quickly (since most people can only tolerate an hour at a time at the most in an MR scanner). Most significantly, the examination could be tailored to answer particular questions in each individual case.

We are only just beginning to realize the potential of functional imaging, which will offer a wealth of information that can be used to improve the service offered to individuals with epilepsy.

Abbreviations

ADC	apparent diffusion coefficient
AMT	α-methyl-L-tryptophan
Asp	aspartate
ATP	adenosine triphosphate
BOLD	blood oxygen level dependent
cBZR	central benzodiazepine receptor
CD	cortical dysplasia
Cho	choline
Cr	creatine
CSI	chemical shift imaging
CT	computed tomography
dwMRI	diffusion-weighted magnetic resonance imaging
EEG	electroencephalogram
EPI	echo planar imaging
FDG	fluoro-deoxyglucose
fMRI	functional magnetic resonance imaging
FMZ	flumazenil
GABA	gamma-aminobutyric acid
Gln	glutamine
Glu	glutamate
Glx	glutamine + glutamate
Hb	hemoglobin
HMPAO	D,L-hexamethylpropyleneamineoxime
HT	hydroxytryptamine
ICS	intracranial stimulation
IED	interictal epileptiform discharge
IGE	idiopathic generalized epilepsy
Ins	inositol
LTLS	lateral temporal lobe seizures
MCD	malformations of cortical development
MR	magnetic resonance
MRI	magnetic resonance imaging
MRS	magnetic resonance spectroscopy
MRSI	magnetic resonance spectroscopy imaging
MTLS	mesial temporal lobe seizures
NAA	N-acetyl aspartate
NGPSE	National General Practice Study of Epilepsy
NMD	neuronal migration disorder
NSE-MRI	National Society of Epilepsy Magnetic Resonance Imaging
PCr	phosphocreatine
PET	positron emission tomography
Pi	inorganic phosphate
ppm	parts per million

SISCOM	subtraction SPECT with coregistration mapping
SMR	standardized mortality rate
SPECT	single photon emission computed tomography
SPM	statistical parametric map
SWS	Sturge–Weber syndrome
Tc	technetium
TS	tuberous sclerosis

Index

BRAIN IMAGING IN SCHIZOPHRENIA
Insights and Applications

Tonmoy Sharma: Institute of Psychiatry, London, UK
Xavier Chitnis: Institute of Psychiatry, London, UK

The application of brain imaging to the study of psychiatric disorders has revolutionized research into the biological basis of schizophrenia. *Brain Imaging in Schizophrenia* provides an overview of the major techniques used in psychiatric neuroimaging, together with a summary of findings from their applications to schizophrenia research. It introduces the major structural and functional imaging modalities used in psychiatry, how these techniques are being used to study schizophrenia, and the impact of neuroimaging on clinical practice.

"...a succinct overview of brain imaging studies in schizophrenia... well illustrated with scan photographs... I would recommend this well-written monograph both to academics and to clinicians."

R Alexander Bantick, *Journal of Neurology, Neurosurgery & Psychiatry*

"This useful little book... outlines with brevity and clarity the basics of each of the principal imaging methods... highly readable...Trainees will find it useful as a primer for exam purposes and old timers a valuable account of where things are."

Prof DG Cunningham, *British Journal of Psychiatry*

Contents:
- Structural brain imaging
- Functional brain imaging
- Structural brain imaging in schizophrenia
- Functional brain imaging in schizophrenia
- Genetics and brain imaging in schizophrenia

Available NOW from all good bookshops and on-line

ISBN: 1 901346 08 0

US$18 / £12.50 / €18

74 pages

MCQS IN CLINICAL RADIOLOGY
A revision guide for the Part 2A FRCR

J Bell: University of British Columbia, Canada
N Davies: The Royal Free Hospital, UK
N Jeyadevan: Royal Marsden Hospital, UK
DM Koh: Royal Marsden Hospital, UK

There are very few radiology multiple choice question books on the market that reflect the current trends and developments in the field of imaging. Hence, the emphasis of this book is on cross-sectional CT and MR imaging. It highlights the current understanding and concepts in the state-of-the-art imaging of a wide range of diseases in the body. The multiple choice questions are organised according to body systems and imaging modalities. There are twelve sections in the book, testing the reader in a broad range of imaging knowledge. The questions are accompanied by expanded answers, which provide the reader with a summary of the key facts relating to a particular topic. This is especially useful in assisting the reader in consolidating his or her understanding of the subject. The questions are devised in a format similar to those encountered in the Part 2A examination of the Royal College of Radiologist (UK) and the Part 2 examination of the Joint Australian and New Zealand College of Radiology. Candidates taking the American Radiology Board examinations will also find the book informative.

Contents:
- Thoracic radiology
- Cardiovascular imaging
- Abdominal imaging
- Uroradiology
- Musculoskeletal imaging
- Neuroradiology
- Head and neck radiology
- Paediatric radiology
- Breast imaging
- Interventional radiology
- Obstetrics and gynaecological imaging
- Nuclear medicine and PET

Available from all good bookshops and on-line from August 2003

ISBN: 1 901346 26 9

US$40 / £25 / €40

200 pages

IMAGING IN STROKE

Editor
Michael Hennerici: University of Heidelberg, Mannheim, Germany

Authors
Julien Bogousslavsky (Switzerland), Gabriel De Freitas (Brazil), Wolf-Dieter Heiss (Germany), Olav Jansen (Germany), Christoph Koch (Germany), Thomas Kucinski (Germany), Joachim Liepert (Germany), Stephen Meairs (Germany), Michael Moseley (Usa), Tobias Neumann-Haefelin (Germany), Fabienne Perren (Switzerland), Cornelius Weiller (Germany), Hermann Zeumer (Germany)

Neuroimaging techniques are crucial in the management of stroke patients. This book is an important resource in the quest to better understand stroke and its heterogeneity. After a first chapter on the classification of stroke, it outlines that the neuroimaging techniques are not only useful to diagnose stroke, its mechanisms and its causes, but are also important for improving our knowledge of the pathophysiology of stroke and its recovery. This book has involved prestigious contributors who have a great knowledge on this topic, and are skilled at describing the current state of knowledge, and also at projecting developments that are likely to occur in the future. This book is useful for all those who have to manage stroke patients at the acute stage, or later, i.e. neurologists, stroke specialists, rehabilitation physicians, and neuroradiologists, and finally for all those who are in search of a focused authoritative review on this subject. It will assume a prominent place as a reference.

"Professor Hennerici and his colleagues provide a clear, beautifully written, cutting edge, and comprehensive overview on what neuroimaging techniques may provide in terms of diagnostic tools and understanding of the pathophysiology of stroke and of its recovery. Its content is of major interest for an optimal management of stroke patients, which requires a sound understanding and an accurate diagnosis."

Didier Leys, University of Lille, France

Contents:
• Introduction
• Classification of stroke
• CT in acute stroke
• MRI in acute stroke
• CTA and MRA in stroke
• Neurosonology in acute stroke
• Intracerebral hemorrhage
• Applications of positron emission tomography in ischemic stroke
• Recovery and plasticity imaging in stroke patients

Available NOW from all good bookshops and on-line

ISBN: 1 901346 25 0

US$45 / £30 / €45

216 pages

STROKE:
Predisposing Conditions

Editor
Didier Leys: University of Lille, France
Foreword by David Sherman: University of Texas Health Science
Center, USA

Authors
Serge Blécic (Belgium), Julien Bogousslavsky (Switzerland), Patrícia Canhão (Portugal), Hugues Chabriat (France), Anna Czlonkowska (Poland), Franz Fazekas (Austria), José Ferro (Portugal), Joost Haan (The Netherlands), Peter Kapeller (Austria), Bengt Karlsson (Sweden), Xavier Leclerc (France), Christian Lucas (France), Jean-Louis Mas (France), Maciej Niewada (Poland), Jean-Pierre Pruvo (France), Marc Reichhart (Switzerland), Reinhold Schmidt (Austria), Emmanuel Touzé (France), Miguel Viana-Baptista (Portugal)

This book is an important resource in our quest to better understand and prevent stroke. It outlines some of the most important, common and rare, factors in the pathogenesis of this disease. As the title implies, stroke cannot be viewed from a narrow perspective. Systemic disorders may be the sole cause or a contributing factor in the genesis of stroke. The contributors have great knowledge of the subject and are skilled at describing our current state of awareness and projecting likely future developments. The discussions are evidence-based and comprehensive, while being focused and concise. The book has utility for both the generalist managing and preventing stroke and for the specialist in search of a focused, up-to-date, authoritative review of the topic. This book will assume a prominent place as a reference and guide for a better understanding and management of stroke.

"Stroke is not a single disease but a complication of one or more different diseases. This book by Professor Leys and colleagues is a beautifully written, cutting-edge and comprehensive, yet succinct, overview of the important common and uncommon causes of ischemic and hemorrhagic stroke. Its contents are pivotal to optimal stroke management, which requires a sound understanding and accurate diagnosis of the underlying cause(s), so that effective (and sometimes risky and costly) acute treatments and secondary prevention strategies can be targeted appropriately to the cause."
Prof Graeme Hankey, Royal Perth Hospital, Australia

Contents:
• Cervical-artery atherosclerosis
• High-risk cardiopathies
• Low-risk cardiopathies
• Cervical-artery dissections
• CADASIL
• Hereditary cerebral amyloid angiopathies
• Vascular white matter changes
• Management of risk factors for stroke: influence on stroke prevention
• Cerebral vein and dural sinus thrombosis
• Non-hemorrhagic cerebral arteriovenous malformations
• Systemic disorders predisposing to stroke
• Rare cerebral angiopathies predisposing to stroke

Available NOW from all good bookshops and on-line

ISBN: 1 901346 34 X

US$60 / £40 / €60

192 pages